Clinical Governance

Clinical Governance

Improving the quality of healthcare
for patients and service users

Mary Gottwald and Gail E. Lansdown

McGraw Hill Education

Open University Press

Open University Press
McGraw-Hill Education
McGraw-Hill House
Shoppenhangers Road
Maidenhead
Berkshire
England
SL6 2QL

email: enquiries@openup.co.uk
world wide web: www.openup.co.uk

and Two Penn Plaza, New York, NY 10121-2289, USA

First published 2014

Copyright © Mary Gottwald and Gail E. Lansdown, 2014

A catalogue record of this book is available from the British Library

ISBN-13: 978-0-335-26280-9
ISBN-10: 0-335-26280-5
eISBN: 978-0-335-26281-6

Library of Congress Cataloging-in-Publication Data
CIP data applied for

Typeset by Aptara Inc., India
Printed and bound by CPI Group (UK) Ltd, Croydon, CR0 4YY

Praise for this book

"In this excellent new book on clinical Governance, Mary Gottwald and Gail Lansdown distil down what this complex topic encompasses. They put bones on the individual components and lead the reader easily through the topic, so that he or she ends up with a good understanding of how the system is supposed to function and their individual responsibilities as a clinician, academic, trainer or manager... I wish that I had been able to read a book such as this when I started off. It would have saved me a lot of time and trouble getting my head around all the aspects of this vital topic. Providing a reliable, safe, high quality service is the major challenge for all of us working in health services, so this fine book is very welcome."

Dr Peter Featherstone MPhil, FRCP, Lead for Clinical Governance in Acute
Medicine
Consultant Physician and Honorary Medical Senior Lecturer Portsmouth
Hospitals NHS Trust

"The book has been developed for pre- and post-registration students, but it will appeal to a wider audience, particularly those who want more knowledge of Governance and its antecedents. The outline of Chapters at the start helpfully leads the reader the appropriate section, and within each section the authors attempt to link clinical governance theory to practical examples. This is further emphasised by the use of reflective questions at the end of each chapter. The chapter on Clinical Audit is excellent, and is of use to anyone including medical staff in terms of how Clinical Audit should be conducted.

It is an excellent, easy read journey through all aspects of Clinical Governance and its application to patient experience, safety and effective senses, ultimately quality of care."

Sharon Linter, Director of Quality and Governance/ Executive Nurse, Cornwall
Partnership NHS Foundation Trust

Contents

8   Evaluating quality care through audit   165
    Mary Gottwald and Gail E Lansdown

List of tables

List of figures

Acknowledgements

The authors would like to thank the following individuals for their help during the writing of this book: Louise Collier and Debbie Hempstead for allowing us to use their SWOT analyses; Ed Gottwald for overall support; Patrick Henry for an introduction to Values Based Practice and how this supports Evidence Based Practice; Marion Waite and Dr Louise Stait for their input on Evidence Based Practice; Dr Helen Walthall for an insight into how education and training can be applied to practice. Lastly we would like to thank Eldo Barkhuizen, our copy editor, for his invaluable help in checking our script prior to publication.

Every effort has been made to trace and acknowledge ownership of copyright and to clear permission for material reproduced in this book. The publishers will be pleased to make suitable arrangements to clear permission with any copyright holders whom it has not been possible to contact.

Overview of the book

This text, which will use working examples from practice, is primarily aimed at pre-registration and post-qualifying students studying on programmes such as Adult Nursing, Children's Nursing, Mental Health Nursing, Learning Disability Nursing, Paramedic, Midwifery, Operating Department Practitioners, Occupational Therapy and Physiotherapy. It will also be a useful text for staff new into post as well as staff moving into management, where an understanding of clinical governance is an important aspect of their role.

The idea for this text comes from our teaching experience both in the United Kingdom and Hong Kong at post-qualifying undergraduate level. Our experience suggests that staff (i.e. post-qualifying students) are able to identify areas of practice where the quality of patient care could be improved. However, the assignments that we read consistently highlight that they find it difficult to take this one step further and are challenged in their learning and ability to apply the clinical governance theories and strategies to their practice.

The rationale for this book

In the UK there have been a number of notorious situations where the quality of patient care has been called into question. Cases such as Beverley Allitt and Harold Shipman initially highlighted the need for well-defined clinical governance structures. Allitt, a State Enrolled Nurse, and Shipman, a doctor, were both serial killers who were convicted of murdering and attempting to murder children (in the case of Allitt) and adults (in the case of Shipman). It was from situations such as these that the National Health Service (NHS) had to review the quality improvement processes to ensure that standards and quality patient care were achieved and this led to the implementation of clinical governance strategies. Whilst Allitt and Shipman triggered early thinking about clinical governance, high profile cases continue to be reported, for example Mid Staffordshire NHS Foundation Trust high mortality rates in Accident and Emergency (AandE), the Banbury nurse jailed in 2006 and the outbreak of *Clostridium difficile* in Maidstone in which 90 patients (definitely or probably) died in 2007.

The aims of this book are

1. To provide readers with a text about clinical governance that is accessible and easy to read
2. To introduce students and practitioners to the practicalities of clinical governance

3. To enable practitioners to apply clinical governance theory and strategies to their practice
4. To show how best clinical governance practice can be applied to internationally common quality issues.

Structure of the book

Each chapter follows the same format. Learning objectives are stated followed by a short introduction that will be given to explain the contents. In most chapters key points and resources will be identified; in all chapters activities will be included to guide reflection. At the end of each chapter, key points and implications for practice will be listed and finally some questions will be posed. The suggested answers to these questions are given in the appendix.

Chapter 1

This chapter commences with a definition of clinical governance to help contextualize five issues that had a negative impact on the quality of service provision in the UK National Health Service. The government's response to these high profile cases together with their 10 year quality improvement programme using clinical governance is outlined. Clinical governance and quality is further defined and critiqued and the preferred definition of clinical governance is given. Finally this chapter considers the engagement and involvement of service users/patients, carers and the public in the provision and improvement of healthcare.

Chapter 2

This theoretical chapter sets the scene for quality issues that occur within practice both locally and internationally. It focuses on the incidence, morbidity and mortality of seven quality issues that impact psychologically on patients/service users and financially on organizations. The examples are taken from a variety of settings and include needle stick injuries, hospital acquired infections, Ventilator Associated Pneumonia, violence, bullying and aggression, pressure ulcers, medication errors and falls in the elderly.

Chapter 3

This chapter begins by exploring how quality circles could be used to help health and social care teams initiate discussions around the quality of care provided. It explores and critiques a number of tools that could be used to analyse the reasons why particular quality issues and poor standards of healthcare arise in practice. These tools are applied to specific examples from practice.

The tools in question are

- Maxwell 6
- 3 organizational dimensions
- Ishikawa's fishbone
- SWOT
- PESTLE.

Chapter 4

This chapter highlights some of the challenges and obstacles impacting on change and discusses how change agents, advocacy groups, involvement of patients and service users can ensure the smooth transition of change. There are a plethora of change management models and this chapter considers

- the Diffusion of Innovation
- Lewin's Force-Field Analysis
- the RAID model
- four A's of change.

Chapter 5

The focus of this chapter is on education and training – one of the key clinical governance strategies. Clinical governance and continuous quality improvement (CQI) can only be successful if healthcare organizations value their staff by having structures in place. These structures are essential to empower clinical and non-clinical staff to engage in education and training.

Concepts of lifelong learning and continued professional development are explored as well as the need for cultural change within health and social care organizations. VARK is discussed as a means to understanding one's own learning style, and practical suggestions on how education and training must be included at the individual, team and organizational level are considered. The chapter concludes with a discussion on learning organizations, organizational culture and makes links to education and training.

Chapter 6

This chapter focuses on the importance of both Evidence Based Practice (EBP) and Values Based Practice (VBP) and how these are applied to clinical governance. Also discussed is the link between EBP and integrated care pathways and care bundles.

Chapter 7

This chapter focuses on the four approaches to quality:

1. Quality control (QC)
2. Total quality management (TQM)
3. Quality assurance (QA)
4. Continuous quality improvement (CQI).

Two further clinical governance strategies are considered, that is, risk management and complaints management. The similarities between risk management and quality assurance are discussed together with complaints management and shared governance.

Chapter 8

This chapter begins with a brief comparison of audit and research, which links to the discussion on Evidence Based Practice in chapter 7. It focuses on how audit can be used to identify where there is a lack of quality care but also provide evidence on excellent care provision. However, it is important to recognize that EBP and audit have different functions. Three validated audit tools are given together with a protocol for designing audit, and the audit cycle with prompts is discussed. Advantages, disadvantages and barriers to audit are outlined. Finally this chapter considers a variety of approaches that teams and individuals might consider.

1

Clinical governance: the context

Mary Gottwald and Gail E Lansdown

Chapter contents

- Learning objectives
- Introduction
- Working definition of clinical governance
- The birth of clinical governance
- Impact of poor care
- The government response
- Government White Papers and reports
- Defining clinical governance
- The framework of clinical governance
- Defining quality
- Linking quality and clinical governance
- Engagement of patients/service users
- Key point summary
- Implications for practice
- End-of-chapter questions
- References

Learning objectives

By the end of this chapter, the reader will be better able to

- understand the rationale for implementing a clinical governance framework
- define concepts such as quality and clinical governance

- critique definitions of quality and clinical governance
- understand the importance of engaging and involving service users, carers and the public in the development of health and social care provision.

Introduction

To begin with a definition of clinical governance will be provided to contextualize five issues that had a negative impact on the quality of service provision in the UK National Health Service. The government's response to these high profile cases together with their ten year quality improvement programme using clinical governance will be outlined. Clinical governance and quality will be further defined and critiqued and the preferred definition of clinical governance will be given. Finally this chapter will consider the engagement and involvement of service users/patients, carers and the public in the provision and improvement of healthcare.

Working definition of clinical governance

The first and well-known definition of clinical governance came from the Department of Health (1998:33): 'A framework through which organisations are accountable for continuously improving the quality of services and safeguarding high standards of care by creating an environment in which clinical care will flourish.'

The birth of clinical governance

A number of high profile damaging incidents have occurred in the UK, some of which are outlined in figure 1.1.

The Bristol Royal Infirmary

Identified that over a ten-year period from 1984 to 1995 the care of children who required complex cardiac surgery was compromised and the mortality rate was approximately double the national average.

Dr Harold Shipman

He was a respected General Practitioner from Hyde in Greater Manchester who over a period of 24 years was thought to be responsible for murdering in the region of 215 patients between 1972 and 1998. Following a trial he was charged with 15 counts of murder.

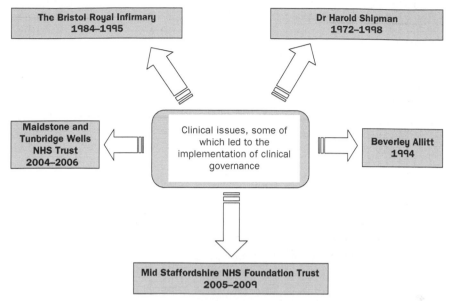

Figure 1.1 Examples of poor quality care. (Adapted from MacDonald 1996, Secretary of State for Health 2001, Department of Health 2006, Healthcare Commission 2007, Francis Report 2013)

Nurse Beverely Allitt

Allitt was employed as a junior nurse on the paediatric ward at Grantham and Kesteven General Hospital and between February and April 1991 she injured eight children; murdered four and was also found guilty of another four counts of attempted murder of children whilst in her care. She was diagnosed with Munchhausen Syndrome by Proxy.

Maidstone and Tunbridge Wells NHS Trust

Between 2004 and 2006 at least 90 patients died from *Clostridium difficile* due to lack of infection prevention and control procedures.

Mid Staffordshire NHS Foundation Trust

Between 2005 and 2009, there was a failure to provide high standards of care, which led to patients being put at risk. Higher mortality rates were reported and there was a public outcry by patients and relatives (CURE the NHS) who experienced poor quality care, for example patients being left in soiled bedding, not being helped at meal times, privacy and dignity not being respected, lack of compassion and candour from staff.

Impact of poor care

Although a number of significant events occurred in the UK that ultimately led to the implementation of clinical governance (figure 1.1), staff commitment is not called into question in any of the above incidences. As identified by the Francis Report (2013), the problem is generally a lack of leadership, ineffective communication, poor organization and teamwork and a lack of means for assessing the quality of care.

The UK Department of Health (2000:11) identified that '10% of inpatient adverse events resulted in harm to patients and approximately half of these errors were avoidable'. At this point litigation claims between 1998 and 1999 from adverse events cost the NHS approximately £400 million. The effects of experiencing poor quality care and going through a litigation process had an impact on service users/patients and staff's physical, emotional and psychological well-being. This would appear to be an ineffective use of public money and supports the need to implement a quality improvement programme through clinical governance.

The government response

The government responded to each of the high profile cases outlined above (see figure 1.2).

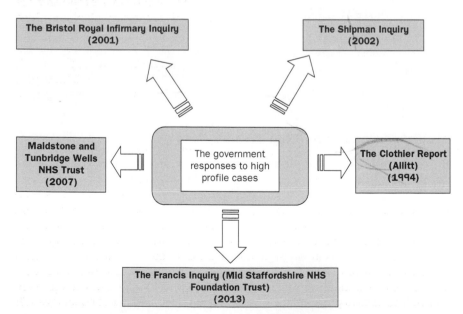

Figure 1.2 Government responses to these incidents.

The Bristol Royal Infirmary Inquiry (2001)

The public inquiry was the largest investigation into medical standards of care in the NHS at that time, and was conducted between 1991 and 2001 and divided into two phases. Phase 1 focused on the events in Bristol and phase 2 focused on the future. The report contained nearly 200 recommendations including better identifying the needs of very sick children, the safety arrangements for caring for very sick children, the competence of healthcare professionals (and their terms of employment to ensure equity between consultants, nurses and managers), standards of care, openness and monitoring of clinical performance, improved leadership and teamwork.

Beverley Allitt and the Clothier Report (1994)

Due to Allitt's psychological disorder, the central responsibility lay with Allitt. However, the report identified failures of management and communications within the hospital. Both the School of Nursing and the Occupational Health Department within the hospital knew of her psychiatric disturbance and yet she was still employed to work in a paediatric unit.

The Shipman Inquiry (Smith 2002)

The Shipman Inquiry was set up in January 2001 as a result of Shipman's conviction in 2000 for the murder of 15 of his patients. A total of six reports were published. The first and last reports examined Shipman's criminal activities as a General Practitioner (GP). The other reports examined the processes and systems that failed to identify his activities (the second report looked at Greater Manchester police, the third report the coroner's system, the fourth report the safe and appropriate use of controlled drugs and the fifth report looked at monitoring and disciplining GPs, whistle-blowing and handling complaints in the NHS).

Maidstone and Tonbridge Wells NHS Trust (2007)

The Healthcare Commission carried out an investigation between 2006 and 2007 to look at the outbreaks of *Clostridium difficile*. The Trust had a relatively high rate of infection and this doubled in the autumn of 2005, although this was not acknowledged at the time. It was identified that the guidelines for management of patients with *Clostridium difficile* did not highlight the importance of isolation of patients with infection. The infection control team were aware of this but there were not enough side rooms available and therefore patients with *Clostridium difficile* were nursed on open wards. The Trust's policy on responding to outbreaks was not considered fit for purpose.

The Francis Report (Mid Staffordshire NHS Foundation Trust) (2013)

This report identified a number of warning signs such as an organizational culture that did not focus on patients (organizational culture will be discussed in more depth in chapter 5), a culture that focused on positive information about the service rather than issues that were causing concern. The inquiry findings showed that staff were too tolerant of poor standards that put patients at risk; there was a failure to communicate between those who had concerns; that monitoring performance management or intervention was someone else's responsibility and there was also an impact of repeated organizational changes. Once again a number of recommendations were made (290 recommendations in total). The key recommendations were a single regulator for financial and care quality, more power to suspend or prosecute hospital boards and individuals, a duty of candour, gagging clauses to be banned in policies and contracts, only registered healthcare professionals should care for patients, clearer leadership to ensure clarity of who is in overall charge of patient's care, complaints to be published on hospital websites and General Practitioners should monitor their patients receiving secondary care.

Government White Papers and reports

Table 1.1 summarizes some of the key government White Papers and reports prior to a more in-depth discussion.

Not only did the government set up inquiries to deal with each of the critical incidents outlined above, but they also published a number of government White Papers in which the recommendations were enshrined.

It was after the recognized high paediatric mortality rates in Bristol and the deaths caused by Beverley Allitt and Dr Harold Shipman that the UK Department of Health White Paper 'The New NHS, Modern, Dependable' (1997) began to address the need to improve the quality of healthcare. The following year 'A First Class Service: Quality in the New NHS' (1998) outlined the then government's strategy for ensuring quality care was provided for all.

These papers identified a 10-year programme that would have quality at the centre of the National Health Service and would lead to guaranteed national standards of excellence. The aim of this quality service would mean that healthcare professionals would be 'doing the right things, at the right time, for the right people, and doing them right – first time' (Department of Health 1997:part 3).

It was at this point that a system of clinical governance in all NHS Trusts was introduced in order to guarantee patient safety and quality care with 'a formal responsibility for quality . . . placed on every health organisation in the country through arrangements for clinical governance at local level' (Department of Health 2000:1). Briefly, clinical governance is an 'organisational concept' (Department of Health 2000:2) that facilitates a system for ensuring

Table 1.1 Government reports and organizations

The New NHS, Modern, Dependable (Department of Health 1997)	The government's response to Allitt, Shipman and the Bristol paediatric cardiac mortality rates. Introduction of clinical governance that focused on improving the quality of healthcare.
A First Class Service: Quality in the New NHS (Department of Health 1998)	This outlined the government's strategy for ensuring quality care was provided to all.
An Organization with a Memory (Department of Health 2000)	A report from an expert group on learning from adverse events in the NHS.
High Quality Care for All: NHS Next Stage Review (Final Report) (Darzi 2008)	A review of the reforms since 1997 and 1998.
National Institute for Clinical Excellence (NICE)	First established in 1997 primarily to provide clinicians with evidence based guidelines for the provision of care (National Service Frameworks). Darzi (2008) recommended that the remit of NICE (now renamed National Institute for Health and Care Excellence) be increased to include the setting of independent standards.
Commission for Health Improvement (CHI)	Established in 1997. One of the key responsibilities of CHI was to monitor and review local clinical governance provisions.
Care Quality Commission (CQC)	Established in 2000 from the merger of the CHI, the Mental Health Act Commission and the Commission for Social Care. The remit is to ensure that national standards are met through monitoring and regulation of health and adult social care services in England.

good quality patient care in which organizations were at that time expected to establish quality improvement programmes. These programmes included audit, clinical risk reduction programmes and processes that identified good practice as well as poor clinical performance. It was also anticipated that organizations would have procedures in place so that adverse events and patient complaints could be quickly identified, investigated, resolved and lessons learned (Department of Health 1997, Department of Health 1998, Department of Health 2000). As Chief Executives had ultimate responsibility for ensuring services were of high quality, monthly and annual reports on clinical governance and the standards of quality of care achieved were to be submitted to

Trust boards, ensuring that clinical governance was as high on the agenda as financial governance.

In order for clinical governance strategies to be successfully implemented, continuing professional development (CPD) became crucial for healthcare staff (CPD will be explored in more depth in chapter 7). Staff were therefore expected to engage in professional development workshops which facilitated leadership skills as well as an understanding of the application of clinical governance strategies (Department of Health 1997). It was also recognized that developments within technology and demographics were changing exponentially and therefore learning had to become 'lifelong' and a continuous process (Sullivan and Garland 2010). The reader is referred to chapter 5, where education and training are discussed in more depth.

Clinical Governance Committees were established and Clinical Governance Leads were appointed within UK hospital Trusts as a result of government directives. These individuals were senior clinicians who became responsible for ensuring that structures and processes were in place and their effectiveness continually monitored (Department of Health 1998).

These Department of Health papers guaranteed that a number of national structures were established to ensure that quality of care was effective, efficient and of a high standard. The two key organizations were

1. NICE (National Institute for Clinical Excellence), established in 1997
2. The Commission for Health Improvement (CHI).

NICE

NICE (now known as The National Institute for Health and Care Excellence) provides healthcare practitioners with specific evidence based guidelines, for example National Service Frameworks on a variety of conditions such as cancer care, children, chronic obstructive pulmonary disease, diabetes, coronary heart disease, older people, mental health, long-term conditions and long-term neurological conditions.

CHI

One of the key responsibilities of CHI was to monitor and review local clinical governance provisions and to support and provide advice on how to ameliorate and prevent adverse events (Department of Health 1998, Department of Health 2000).

The Prime Minister at the time, Gordon Brown, asked Lord Darzi, Junior Health Minister and a practising surgeon, to suggest a strategy to meet the health needs of Londoners. The report, *Healthcare for London: A Framework for Action*, was published in July 2007. Darzi was also asked to review the reforms achieved since the Department of Health 1997 and 1998 White Papers. Furthermore he collaborated with patients and staff to identify a vision for the development and future of the health service in the twenty-first century. In his report *High Quality Care for All: NHS Next Stage Review (Final Report)* (2008:2), Darzi envisioned that the UK would have 'an NHS that gives patients and the public more information and choice, works in partnership and has quality of care at its heart'.

Darzi (2008) recommended that the remit of NICE was to be increased to include the setting of more independent quality standards. Additionally a new National Quality Board would give clear advice to ministers on the priority of those clinical standards. Key priorities focused on the provision of safe and effective quality care but also on ensuring that the patient's experience of care was good. This is endorsed by the Royal College of Nursing (RCN) who state on their website that the main focus of clinical governance is to improve the patient experience (Scrivener 2010). Scrivener is an information manager on the RCN's quality improvement programme.

Care Quality Commission

Following this in 2009, the Commission for Health Improvement (CHI), the Mental Health Act Commission and the Commission for Social Care were amalgamated to become the Care Quality Commission (CQC). The key aim of the CQC is to ensure that national standards are met through monitoring and regulation of health and adult social care services in England. NHS organizations and social care providers now have to register with the Care Quality Commission. The Care Quality Commission is a self-governing watchdog that audits and regulates establishments, namely hospitals, dentists, ambulances, care homes and services in people's own homes and elsewhere against a framework of standards to ensure that national standards of quality and safety are met. These standards include basic needs such as

- guaranteeing service users have the right food and liquid
- the environment is clean and safe
- to ensure that patients and services users are involved in their care and dignity and respect are safeguarded
- and to ensure that staff have the required skills and knowledge and that the quality of services is regularly audited (Care Quality Commission).

Clinical Commissioning Groups

From April 2013, Clinical Commissioning Groups (CCGs) have replaced Primary Care Trusts and one of their key aims will be to meet patient needs through providing the 'right care, right place, first time' (Department of Health 2012a:6). The NHS Commissioning Board also includes this statement in their vision for 'ensuring we have the right staff, with the right skills in the right place' (Department of Health 2012b:22). It is evident that quality care remains on the national agenda, although recent events in 2012–2013 (Francis Report

2013) suggest that there has been limited progress, since the phrase ensuring we have 'the right staff with the right skills in the right place' (Department of Health 2012a:22) is a repetition of the phrase 'doing the right things, at the right time, for the right people, and doing them right – first time' (Department of Health 1997:part 3).

Key points

- The Department of Health is committed to improving the quality of healthcare.
- Staff need to review practice continuously in order to meet national standards of care.
- Clinical governance remains on the national agenda.

Defining clinical governance

Activity

- Before reading the definitions below, write down four key words that you feel could be included in a definition of clinical governance. It will be interesting to see how your ideas link to the definitions.

The literature presents a number of definitions for us to consider. Firstly, 'A framework through which organisations are accountable for continuously improving the quality of services and safeguarding high standards of care by creating an environment in which clinical care will flourish' (Department of Health 1998:33).

According to Lugon (2005), healthcare professionals should incorporate clinical governance strategies into everyday practice, and one of the important things to note from the definition above (*creating an environment*) is that clinical governance is relevant to both staff and patients; therefore the environment impacts on both staff and patients. For example, the quality of patient care could be affected if staff work in an environment in which support or opportunities to develop their knowledge and skills is lacking. Lack of resources (low staffing levels, equipment and medication) could also impact on both staff and patients. From the patient's viewpoint, admission to a mixed ward could affect their overall experience and their perception of quality care.

A second definition to consider: 'Clinical Governance places a duty on all health professionals, clinicians and managers to ensure that the level of clinical service they deliver to patients is satisfactory, consistent and responsive' (Swage 2004:4).

Although cited in Swage (2004), the ideas for this definition stem from the Department of Health (1997) White Paper 'The New NHS Modern Dependable'. This definition reinforces the need for all healthcare professionals, whether clinicians or managers, to be accountable for the service they provide to patients. The National Service Frameworks are one of the systems designed to support staff to do this. Swage (2004:5) suggests that clinical governance is an 'umbrella under which all aspects of quality can be continually monitored and it needs to be led by clinicians'.

A final definition to consider is that of Som (2004:89):

A governance system for healthcare organisations that promotes an integrated approach towards management of inputs, structures and processes to improve the outcome of the healthcare service delivery where health staff work in an environment of greater accountability for clinical quality.

One of the strengths of Som's definition is that he encapsulates and reinterprets the two Department of Health definitions, and in so doing captures the complexity of the issue. As well as considering the *environment* (Department of Health 1998) and *accountability* (Swage 2004) he also discusses inputs, structure, processes and outcome and each of these are aligned with clinical governance (table 1.2). All of these concepts will be discussed and applied to practice in later chapters.

Table 1.2 Attributes of clinical governance (Som's 2004 definition)

Inputs	Includes financial resources, human resources, infrastructure and policy (where quality is a legislative requirement of the organization).
Structure	Includes the requirement to provide education and training and continuing professional development (CPD), guidelines for clinical care, for example integrated care pathways, clinical risk management, promoting evidence based medicine (Evidence Based Practice), audit and leadership development. The Chief Executive Officer (CEO) is made accountable for the standard of care provided.
Processes	Includes the implementation of risk management, education and training, leadership development, audit and management of patient information (confidentiality and anonymity). It also includes processes to record 'near misses' and adverse events.
Outcomes	Includes continuous quality improvements (CQI), patient satisfaction and reduced number of 'near misses' and adverse events. Better rapport between patients and clinicians and improved collaboration between professionals and managers are also stressed. Additionally interventions being supported through Evidence Based Practice are included (further discussed in chapter 7).

Activity

- Have another look at the four key words that you wrote at the beginning of this section. Have they changed and, if so, why?
- Which is your preferred definition?
- Why do you prefer one definition more than the others?

Using Som's four organizational dimensions (see figure 1.3), analyse the incidents discussed at the beginning of this chapter to see where the problems arose in relation to input, structure, process and outcome.

The questions below will help to guide your thinking.

Input:

- Did financial, human or environmental resources lead to the incident?

Structure:

- Was a clear education and training programme available?
- Were guidelines for clinical care evident?
- Was there a failure with leadership?

Processes:

- What processes were in place? Risk management? Leadership development? Implementation of education and training and the recording of 'near misses' and adverse events?

Outcome:

- How did the above impact on the outcome? For example, CQI, patient satisfaction and improved communication and collaboration and reduced number of 'near misses'?

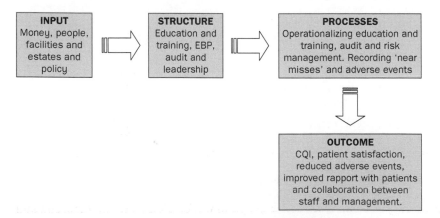

Figure 1.3 Four organizational dimensions (Som 2004)

The framework of clinical governance

The definition of clinical governance presented by the Department of Health (1998) states that clinical governance is a 'framework', and, as previously discussed, Swage (2004:5) states that clinical governance 'provides an umbrella under which all aspects of quality can be gathered and continuously monitored' but what does this involve? Figure 1.4 illustrates this more clearly. Clinical governance is the overarching framework and can be implemented through each strategy on the 'spokes' of this umbrella. It can be seen that some of the spokes of the umbrella (figure 1.4) link to Som's organizational dimensions outlined above.

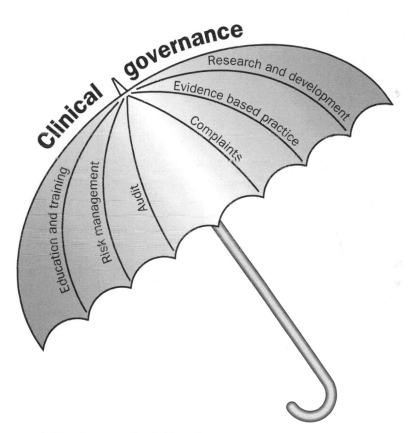

Figure 1.4 The framework of clinical governance.

The strategies discussed in later chapters will be aligned to the umbrella and Som's (2004) organizational dimensions.

Defining quality

Quality is a personal construct dependent on one's beliefs and values and therefore quality could be considered to link to one's perception. Moullin (2003:13) defines quality succinctly as 'fitness for purpose' but one could then question what this means. If each organization set their own standards and 'purpose', then it could be perceived that the quality of care would vary and the impact of this could be that quality of care could be poor in some organizations. Ovretveit (1990, cited in Moullin 2003:14) provides a more in-depth definition: 'Fully meeting the needs of those who need the service most, at the lowest cost to the organisation, within limits and directives set by higher authorities.'

According to Darzi (2008:2), quality is defined as 'clinically effective, personal and safe', and for Birnbaum and Van Buren (2010:81) quality can be seen as a 'journey not a destination'. This last definition is useful for organizations to remember because in order to achieve successful outcomes, quality must continuously be improved through constantly developing inputs, structures and process (Som 2004).

Whatever definition of quality is used, there needs to be an understanding between the organization and service users, carers and the public.

Linking quality and clinical governance

Quality is of interest to various people both internal and external to health and social care organizations, for example groups or 'stakeholders' such as patients, relatives, government and hospital staff. They have an interest in healthcare, they deliver healthcare, and/or are held responsible for the clinical effectiveness of service delivery. *Clinical governance* aims to put the delivery of *clinical quality* at the centre of healthcare provision. It should be evidence based, widely shared, using skilled staff and appropriate facilities.

Clinical governance includes (see figure 1.5) implementing *Evidence Based Practice* (as suggested by Som 2004) into everyday patient care to ensure that healthcare professionals know what they are doing works and why it works. It includes *continuous quality improvement* (CQI) so that healthcare professionals always aim to improve practice, guarantee that risks are managed, and learning from incidents and accidents is shared. Shared learning

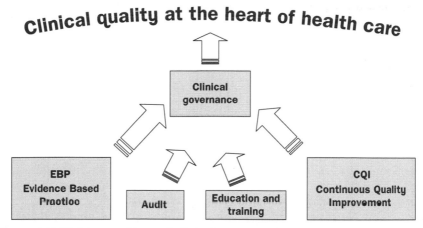

Figure 1.5 Linking quality and clinical governance.

(education and training) ensures that healthcare professionals aim to prevent what mistakes they can, limit what they cannot prevent and most importantly learn from mistakes that are made and to prevent them happening again in the future. Finally clinical governance includes clinical *audit* to assess compliance and to encourage reflection on individual and team work; checking to see if what should happen is happening

Engagement of patients/service users

The birth of patient/service user engagement

Since its inception in 1948, the NHS has changed and continues to change, and after the high profile cases discussed earlier it became essential to re-establish trust in the NHS. The NHS is funded through public taxation and therefore service users, carers and the general public are in the main interested in the standard of care provided. These groups increasingly want to be given the opportunity to be involved and have a say in how healthcare services are developed in the future (Haxby et al. 2010). Additional to this is the ready access to the internet, which has enabled service users to be more knowledgeable about their health and therefore what they expect a healthcare service to provide. Darzi (2008) strongly acknowledged this importance of putting service users at the centre of healthcare. Following the Darzi report, service users began to be involved in decision-making in relation to where they received their care package, for example in which hospital they would wish to receive secondary care and also in determining the level of care they could expect. This involvement of service users in decision-making has helped to reduce medical paternalism.

Definitions of patient/service user engagement

According to Haxby et al. (2010:314) service user involvement is defined as:

> individual involvement (for example, the central role of patients in decisions about their own health and care) and involvement at a more collective level (patient representatives, for example actively contributing to NHS policy and planning decisions).

Instead of 'service user involvement', the Care Quality Commission use the term 'patient and public engagement'. The CQC runs an 'Acting Together' programme within England, which involves discussions with 'experts by experience', that is, those who have first-hand experience of health and social care services thus ensuring that the voices of service users are heard. These experts are very much part of the CQC in that they are part of the inspections that take place and they are also included in process development activities within the CQC. During the unannounced visits, the CQC provide the 'experts' with topics they would like discussed and then the 'experts' independently talk to residents in care homes and/or patients in hospitals to find out their viewpoints on what organizations are doing well and what could be improved upon. Any concerns are then reported back to the CQC inspector.

Rationale for engagement

One of the key reasons for engaging service users and carers is because the recipients of care have an understanding of specific interventions. Ultimately they are experienced and have ideas on how a service needs to be developed to ensure continuous quality improvement. Healthcare professionals may feel that their knowledge and expertise are being challenged (medical paternalism). However, gaining an understanding of the service user's perspective will benefit future provision and improve patient care.

Redesign versus co-design

Bate and Robert (2007:27) go further and state that the above is not enough: 'The role of users and the value and justification for their being there is to bring the knowledge of their experience to the table so that the designers can work with them to translate and build that knowledge into new and future designs.'

Bate and Robert (2007), conclude that rather than redesigning the system around the patient, the service could be co-designed with the patient. This is further supported by Gehry (2003), who states that 'without the client, you're one hand, you're the sound of one hand clapping. The client is the variable, and if the client engages with you, that's the opportunity' (Gehry 2003, cited in Bate and Robert 2007:16). Although Gehry (2003) is speaking from an architectural perspective, his thoughts echo those of Bate and Robert (2007).

Level of engagement

Following the Darzi Report (2008), it is now widely agreed that service users need to be involved and engaged at a variety of levels within healthcare organizations, for example at Board level, Committee level and at an individual level (Bond and Magill 2010). This involvement has led to the need for increased communication and greater collaboration, so that service users can have a positive impact on decisions and that their presence is not simply tokenistic. This could be seen as 'adding value' both to professionals and to service users (Bond and Magill 2010).

Organizations must ensure that the improvement of quality care is continuous (continuous quality improvement) and, as Haxby et al. (2010) highlight, this also means that service users must be engaged in constant discussions and plans; in other words their involvement is not a 'one off event'. Whilst healthcare professionals have an understanding of the evidence base of care, it is the recipients who have an understanding of the experience and so through working together there is a better chance of standards, as set out in the National Service Frameworks, being raised and the expectations of both the professionals and service users being met.

Activity

- How are service users included in the delivery of their care in your workplace?
- Thinking about your workplace and Bate and Robert's (2007) suggestion, are service users involved in *redesigning* the service around the patient or *co-designing* the service with the patient? If the former, how might this be changed?

Practice examples

Another aspect to consider is that the service user's priorities may differ from that of the professional.

This is illustrated in my early career as an occupational therapist, working on a stroke rehabilitation ward. As an occupational therapist a priority of mine was to facilitate patients to be able to dress themselves independently. One of my patients explained to me that although they could get dressed without any assistance, it would take hours and leave them exhausted, so they would prefer to employ someone to dress them. By paying someone it enabled this patient to spend their time engaged more purposively in their hobbies. This illustrates how my priorities were different from the patient's.

Bond and Magill (2010:330) identify other examples where priorities between the professional and service user differ. Firstly an individual whose hobby was fishing prioritized resolving his incontinence problem first before other multiple problems. By having his incontinence problem resolved it meant he could spend the day fishing without any embarrassments.

Secondly a Muslim patient wished to have the osteoarthritis in his knees dealt with prior to other problems, to enable him to kneel to pray. This person spent a number of hours each week praying in the local mosque and being able to kneel without pain had become the main priority.

These examples illustrate how service users are being involved at a micro or personal level with *co-designing* their healthcare. Bate and Robert (2007) would take this further to empower service users to *co-design* the service at a macro level.

Having discussed the importance of establishing relationships and partnerships between service users and healthcare providers it is important to consider how service users can be involved.

Methods of engagement

Activity

- Write a list of the different methods that could be used to involve service users in planning and co-designing healthcare services in your own area of practice.

Some suggestions are provided below which may be similar to the ones you identified in your answer to the above activity. Chapter 3 will discuss another process that could be used through setting up quality circles.

Service users/'experts by experience' can become involved with clinical governance through surveys that are distributed in order to gain an understanding of their perceptions. Surveys collect quantitative data; for example through using likert scales. For a more in-depth understanding, qualitative methods could be used, such as one-to-one interviews. However, this could be a daunting experience for the service user who may see the professional as being someone in a position of power and therefore they may feel intimidated and not want to give their true opinion. One way to overcome this is to engage service users/'experts by experience', in focus groups. One advantage of using focus groups is that a number of individuals (6–8) could be included in discussions at the same time and so individuals may feel more comfortable about sharing their opinions (Sale 2005, Wright and Hill 2003).

Patient Voices Programme

This programme offers service users/patients a very different opportunity from the above method of using surveys and interviews. One of the key aims of the Patient Voices Programme is to put patients 'at the heart of healthcare' (Department of Health 2008) to facilitate collaboration between healthcare professionals and patients to work together to continue to develop patient care. Initially the Patient Voices were funded by the NHS Clinical Governance Support Team (Patient Voices Programme).

Patient Voices are short digital stories using a variety of media, such as video and audio recordings or music. These stories allow individuals to share their experiences and feelings on what it was like to be on the receiving end of healthcare and these are then shared with hospital Trust Boards and teams. As well as providing examples of excellent care, digital stories could provide a number of examples of poor care, such as 'near misses', poor access to care or negative staff attitudes.

Evidence from Manchester Mental Healthcare Trust shows that these stories enable strategy planners and frontline staff to practice in a more informed and compassionate manner and as a result complaints in relation to care and staff attitudes have reduced.

Key point

- The Patient Voices Programme encourages partnership working between healthcare professionals and service users and could be deemed to be less frightening and more productive than interviews or questionnaires.

Key point summary

In this chapter we have considered the historical perspective and the clinical issues that led to the inception of the concept of organizational clinical governance. Clinical governance is an overarching framework under which various structures and processes sit (Som 2004), thereby ensuring that the quality of healthcare is continuously improved.

Collaboration and partnership working between health and social care staff and the service users/'experts by experience' who have first-hand experience of healthcare is recommended. Also recommended is the notion of involving service users/'experts by experience' in co-design of the service rather than redesign of their care (Bate and Robert 2007).

- Clinical governance is a framework used to improve the quality of care provided.
- Clinical governance relates to both staff and service users.
- All staff employed within health and social care are accountable for the standards of care provided.
- For quality care provision to be successful, patient and public engagement and involvement is essential.

Implications for practice

* Healthcare organizations must ensure that all healthcare staff, service users and the public are involved in the development of the quality of care.
* Shared learning and candour should be part of an organization's ethos.
* A shared leadership approach supports clinical governance.
* Two-way communication is essential to minimize adverse clinical incidents.

End-of-chapter questions

1. How does an understanding of the definitions of clinical governance help you develop your practice?
2. Knowing that clinical governance is everyone's responsibility, how could you become more proactive in implementing your organization's strategy for quality improvement?
3. What is the role of the clinical governance lead in your organization?
4. How do you feed into this role?

See the Appendix on page 191 for suggested answers to these questions.

References

Bate P and Robert G (2007) *Bringing user experience to healthcare improvement: The concepts, methods and practices of experience-based design.* Oxford: Radcliffe Publishing

Birnbaum D and Van Buren J (2010) Applying continuous improvement in public reporting: What should government reports do for quality improvement? *Clinical Governance: An International Journal,* 15 (2), 79–91

Bond J and Magill J (2010) Patient and public involvement (PPI) in Haxby E, Hunter D and Jaggar S (2010) *An introduction to clinical governance and patient safety.* Oxford: Oxford University Press

Bristol Royal Infirmary Inquiry (2001) *The report of the public inquiry into children's heart surgery at the Bristol Royal Infirmary 1984–1995: Learning from Bristol.* Bristol: Bristol Royal Infirmary inquiry

Care Quality Commission http://www.cqc.org.uk/public/about-us (accessed 05.04.2013)

Clothier Report (1997) http://www.cdn.pcc-cic.org.uk/sites/default/files/articles/attach ments/clothier_report_1977.pdf (accessed 04.01.2013)

Darzi (2008) *High quality care for all: NHS next stage review (final report).* London: Department of Health

Department of Health (1997) *The new NHS: Modern, dependable.* Available at http://www.web.archhive.nationalarchives.gov.uk/+/www.dh.gov.uk

Department of Health (1998) *A first class service: Quality in the new NHS.* London: Department of Health

Department of Health (2000) *An organisation with a memory.* London: HMSO

Department of Health (2006) *Good doctors, safer patients: Proposals to strengthen the system to assure and improve the performance of doctors and to protect the safety of patients*. London: Department of Health

Department of Health (2008) *High quality care for all: NHS next stage review final report*. London: HMSO. Available at http://www.official-documents.gov.uk/document/cm74/7432/7432.pdf (accessed 21.01.2014)

Department of Health (2012a) *An organisation with a memory*. London: HMSO

Department of Health (2012b) *Compassion in practice. Nursing, midwifery and care staff. Our vision and strategy*. London: Department of Health

Francis Report (2013) *Report of the Mid Staffordshire NHS Foundation Trust public inquiry*. London: HMSO

Gehry F (2003) *Gehry talks: Architecture and process*. London: Thames and Hudson

Haxby E, Hunter DH and Jaggar S (2010) *An introduction to clinical governance and patient safety*. New York: Oxford University Press.

Healthcare Commission (2007) *Investigation into outbreaks of Clostridium difficile at Maidstone and Tunbridge Wells NHS Trust*. London: Commission for Healthcare Audit

Health Care for London (2007) *A framework for action*. Available at http://www.nhshistory.net/darzilondon.pdf (accessed 20.01.2014)

Lugon M (2005) Clinical governance – from rhetoric to reality. *Current Paediatrics*, 15, 460–465

MacDonald A (1996) Responding to the results of the Beverly Allitt inquiry. *Nursing Times*, Jan 10–6:92 (2), 23–25

Moullin M (2003) *Delivering excellence in health and social care*. Maidenhead: Open University Press

Patient Voices Programme http://www.pilgrimprojects.co.uk (accessed 21.08.13)

Sale D (2005) *Understanding clinical governance and quality assurance: Making it happen*. Basingstoke: Palgrave Macmillan

Scrivener R (2010) Nursing practice issues. Available at http://www.rcn.org.uk (accessed 21.07.2013)

Secretary of State for Health (2001) The report of the public inquiry into children's heart surgery at the Bristol Royal Infirmary 1984–1995. London: Department of Health

Smith Dame J (2002) *The Shipman Inquiry: Death certification and the investigation of deaths by coroners*. Manchester: HMSO

Som C (2004) Clinical governance: A fresh look at its definition. *Clinical Governance: An International Journal*, 9, 87–90

Sullivan E and Garland G (2010) *Practical leadership and management in healthcare: For nurses and allied health professionals*. London: Pearson

Swage T (2004) *Clinical governance in healthcare practice*. London: Butterworth-Heinemann

Wright J and Hill P (2003) *Clinical governance*. London: Churchill Livingstone

2

Quality: the key issues

Gail E Lansdown

Chapter contents

- Learning objective
- Introduction
- Needle stick injuries (NSIs)
- Hospital acquired infections (HAIs)
- Ventilator-acquired pneumonia (VAP)
- Violence, bullying and aggression (VBA)
- Pressure ulcers (PUs)
- Medication errors
- Falls in the elderly
- Key point summary
- Implications for practice
- End-of-chapter questions
- References

Learning objective

By the end of this chapter, the reader will have a better understanding of

- the incidence, morbidity and mortality of a number of quality issues that impact on patient/client care.

Introduction

The previous chapter introduced the concept of clinical governance and its importance in ensuring that standards and quality patient care are continuously monitored and improved. This chapter will focus on the incidence, morbidity and mortality of seven quality issues that impact on patients/service users both locally and internationally. These examples have been taken from a variety of settings. The following chapters will explore the causes of these quality issues and will discuss clinical governance strategies that can be used to improve quality care.

The examples discussed below illustrate incidents that regularly occur and demonstrate how the clinical governance framework may well not have been appropriately implemented by all staff.

Needle stick injuries (NSIs)

Incidence of NSIs

Needle stick injuries occur around the globe, across all staff working within a healthcare environment and in all settings where needles are used.

Even when standard precautions are observed, needle stick injuries (NSIs) are common (Murray 2009). Occupational exposure to pathogenic microbes acquired by a needle stick injury is associated with a small but significant risk to a healthcare professional's career, health, family and patients (Pathak et al. 2012). Most NSIs occur on wards (36%) with the operating theatre the second most common setting (17%) of all high-risk exposures reported to the Health Protection Agency (Health Protection Agency 2008).

In 2004, Elmiyeh et al. carried out a confidential survey at an NHS district general hospital. Three hundred healthcare professionals were asked to complete a questionnaire to elicit their views of NSI and their attitudes to reporting. Completed questionnaires were received from 279 members of staff, of whom 38% had experienced at least one NSI in the past year and 74% had experienced a NSI in their career. Only 51% reported all NSIs, despite 80% of the respondents knowing that such incidents should be reported. Despite a higher chance of causing injury, doctors were less likely to report than nurses.

In 2006, the number of exposure incidents was estimated to be more than 50,000 and under reporting is well documented (Elder and Paterson 2006). Between 1997 and 2008, a total of 3773 blood borne virus exposure incidents involving healthcare workers in the UK were reported to the Health Protection Agency (Health Protection Agency 2008). Of these, 76% were percutaneous injuries mainly to medical and nursing staff, with 9% to ancillary staff. Exposure to Hepatitis C virus infected patients was the greatest, but only 22% of these had follow-up samples collected at the recommended time intervals.

Most of the data on NSIs related to healthcare workers is from hospital settings; however, it has recently been shown that the risk to healthcare workers in community settings is substantial (Gershon et al. 2007).

Thomas and Murray (2009), in their study of needle stick injury in UK surgeons, noted that surgeons often make decisions without observing hospital sharps policy, thus exposing surgeons to unnecessary risk. Of the 98 surgeons in the hospital in question, 77 responded to the questionnaire and 44 reported having had a NSI. Of these 3% stated they had followed the needle stick policy, 70% performed first aid (informing the scrub nurse, changing the needle and gloves) and 21% ignored the NSI and continued to work. Thomas and Murray conclude that NSIs are a common problem among surgeons and are under-reported.

Healthcare workers at Lok Nayak Hospital in New Delhi are required to self-report NSIs, immediately after exposure, by a questionnaire. Of the 376 NSIs reported by healthcare workers, 55.6% were by males, and 47.3% by females. Of those reported, 47% were by interns, 27.08% by residents and 10.1% by staff nurses. Cleaning staff reported 1.1%, suggesting that injuries could also be experienced in the process of waste disposal. A greater percentage was noted in the Medical Department. The percentage of NSIs was 78.2% in wards, 5.9% in the Emergency Department and 5.6% in the Intensive Care Unit (Sharma et al. 2012).

Hiko et al. (2012) in their systematic review of the effectiveness of training to prevent NSI in healthcare professionals report the following:

- NSIs can occur in hospitals, health centres, clinics and in paramedic emergency care.
- More attention has been focused on NSIs since the HIV/AIDS pandemic.
- The WHO (2002) estimated that worldwide 2.5% of HIV cases and 40% of Hepatitis B and C infections among healthcare professionals are through NSIs.
- The commonest route of infection of HIV and Hepatitis B and C from a patient to a healthcare professional is by NSI. The risk of contacting Hepatitis C from a NSI is 1% to 5% (Joint WHO/ILO Guidelines 2005).
- The Health Protection Agency in 2008 reported that nine healthcare practitioners had been infected with Hepatitis C within a six year period, more than 2000 incidents of NSIs were reported with 47% being exposed to Hepatitis C and 26% to HIV. More than a third of the incidents occurred during disposal of sharps with some occurring during attempts to recap needles.
- Blame and stigma are attached to reporting NSIs (Wilburn and Eijkemans 2004).

The incidence of Hepatitis C virus (HCV) infection has been significantly reduced since the introduction of single use medical equipment (Scaggiante et al. 2013). However, they report the case of a 19-year-old student nurse who contracted HCV after recapping a 23-gauge needle after taking blood.

Psychological impact of NSIs

A recent EU directive (Directive 2010/32/EU) on the prevention of NSIs makes brief reference to the requirement for counselling post injury, but does not discuss the psychiatric consequences of NSIs. Whilst the occupational hazard of NSIs is well documented, there are limited studies addressing the psychiatric effects (Green and Griffiths 2013). According to Green and Griffiths, severe psychological pathologies may be exhibited in staff that do not contract a blood borne infection. This is documented in children in the study conducted by Papenburg et al. (2008). In Japan, depressive symptoms have been identified in medical students suffering from NSIs (Wada et al. 2007). Sohn et al. (2006) reported that 71% of healthcare workers had experienced NSIs and had higher scores for anxiety and depression than their colleagues. Also, both studies state that further research is needed in this area. The Health Protection Agency (2008), focusing on a recent UK government report, discussed the possible physical consequences of NSI, but no reference to mood or psychiatric disorders was made (Green and Griffiths 2013).

Green and Griffiths (2013) found that psychiatric disorders in NSI healthcare workers were similar to other post-traumatic stress disorders in severity and lasted for nine months on average. The sample size of their study is small (n = 17), but the cases they describe presented with anxiety associated with a continued perception of unacceptable risk; this anxiety, in the main, did not resolve until definitive blood results had been received. Green and Griffiths' study also showed that several of the participants reported deterioration in their sexual relationships following advice to use barrier contraception, whilst others refrained from sex in order to reduce the risk of transmission to their partner.

Naghavi et al. (2013), with a larger sample size than Green and Griffiths, studied trainee doctors in a university hospital in the UK and found that, of the 147 doctors who participated, 54% had an NSI during their training and, of these, 38% were not reported to Occupational Health or the Emergency Department. This latter point supports previously discussed literature in this chapter. Of doctors who had experienced an NSI, 12% showed evidence of post-traumatic stress disorder (PTSD) in comparison to a 3% prevalence of PTSD in the general population.

Financial Impact of NSIs

NSIs result in a significant financial burden. In California, 903 people (consisting of nurses, orderlies, janitors, maids and doctors) sustained a NSI between 1992 and 2003 with 7% of these leading to more than 31 days of absence from work (Leigh et al. 2008). In the UK, the estimated cost to the National Health Service of NSI through insulin administration alone is £600,000 (Trueman et al. 2008) and litigation is becoming an increasing problem.

Naghavi et al. (2013) highlight not only the psychological impact of NSIs in trainee doctors but further discuss the financial burden related to follow-up testing, treatment and time off work.

Hospital acquired infections (HAIs)

Hospitals, nursing homes and outpatient departments can be dangerous places for the acquisition of a hospital acquired infection (HAI). The most common types of HAI, or nosocomial infection, are surgical wound infection, respiratory infection, genitourinary infection and gastrointestinal infection. Immunocompromised, the elderly and young children are usually the most susceptible and infections are transmitted from hospital staff, poor infection control procedures or droplets from other infected patients. HAIs are common, costly (directly, indirectly and intangibly) and potentially lethal (Klein et al. 2011).

Two HAIs have often been reported in the press: *Clostridium difficile* (*C. difficile*) and methicillin resistant *Staphylococcus aureus* (MRSA).

Methicillin resistant *Staphylococcus aureus* (MRSA)

MRSA is a growing problem. The infection can go undiagnosed for a long period of time and a person may not know he or she is colonized or carrying the infection. Whilst not always life threatening, MRSA is a global cause of morbidity and mortality.

Methicillin was first used in 1959 to treat infections caused by penicillin-resistant *Staphylococcus aureus*, and two years later, in 1961, reports from the UK suggested that *S. aureus* isolates had become resistant to methicillin (Enright et al. 2002). MRSA has a serious financial impact on patients and hospitals (Hudson et al. 2011), and until the 1990s, MRSA mainly infected people with frequent attendance at healthcare facilities (healthcare associated MRSA or HA-MRSA). Hudson et al. (2011) state that the rate of HA-MRSA (symptomatic and asymptomatic) in general hospital populations in the United States is 6–21%, with 9–24% infections in ICUs.

Since the 1990s, however, community-associated MRSA (CA-MRSA) has become more prevalent and causes infection in young children and adults who have not had previous contact with healthcare facilities. CA-MRSA has been reported globally (Wallin et al. 2008) and it is particularly virulent in young children. Some reports suggest that CA-MRSA is being found in hospital settings and that it is becoming more prevalent than HA-MRSA in this setting (D'Agata et al. 2009, Popovich et al. 2013).

The risk factors for acquiring MRSA are many and varied (Gosbell 2004) and include

- chronic dermatoses
- medical illness
- surgery
- attending healthcare facilities
- use of antibiotics
- intravenous lines
- admission to an ICU
- proximity to colonized patients/staff.

Diagnosis in the community (CA-MRSA) is complicated as patients may not have these risk factors.

Not only does MRSA spread quickly from person to person but it also readily contaminates the environment and its containment requires strict infection control measures involving isolating the infected patient, cleaning the environment and punctilious hand hygiene, which can be increased by the use of alcoholic antiseptic hand rubs over antiseptic hand washes.

Psychological impact of acquiring MRSA

Interestingly, Pegues (2013) reminds us of the psychological impact of isolating patients with MRSA, stating that this not only results in decreased patient–healthcare professional contact and thus quality of care and subsequently patient satisfaction, but also an increased possibility of delirium and depression.

Financial impact of MRSA

The study of Macedo-Vinas et al. (2013) conducted at a 2200-bed centre, providing both primary and tertiary care between 1 January and 3 December 2009, showed

- 167 MRSA-infected patients
- 115 colonized but not infected patients
- 25,766 MRSA free patients.

Generally the proportion of patients in medical, surgical and ICU wards was similar.

The crude mean length of stay (LOS) was 37.3, 33.0 and 8.8 days for MRSA-infected patients, colonized but not infected patients and MRSA-free patients respectively. Using a variety of different analytical approaches, they estimated that MRSA infection cost approximately 800 Swiss francs per day.

Clostridium difficile

Clostridium difficile infection (CDI) was identified in 1978 as the cause of pseudomembranous colitis, and has since evolved into an aggressive HAI (Badger et al. 2012).

CDI is an HAI that causes a range of symptoms from diarrhoea to toxic megacolon and death (Hardy et al. 2012), and is generally associated with poor outcomes for patients (Song et al. 2008). The infection is associated with increased healthcare costs as it increases average length of stay, and for every ten patients that acquire CDI in hospital, one patient will die (Forster et al. 2010). It is the most common cause of hospital acquired diarrhoea in the developed world, and, whilst the incidence of the infection has fallen in the UK, it is still a major problem for hospitals (Enoch and Aliyu 2012).

The route of transmission is via the faecal-oral route, although there is now evidence of airborne spread (Best et al. 2010). CDI may be cultured from the stool of healthy adults, but most people remain asymptomatic. It is the use of antibiotics that disrupt the gut flora that typically supports the proliferation of CDI and thus results in infection. A care bundle approach has resulted in a reduction of the number of cases in the UK (Department of Health 2007), and includes the prudent prescription of antibiotics, early isolation of patients, good hand hygiene, the use of personal protective equipment and cleaning of the environment. As antibiotics are seen to be part of the problem and may predispose a patient to CDI, it is important to implement guidelines for the appropriate use of antibiotics, and broad-spectrum antibiotics should be avoided.

Wenisch et al. (2012) compared 185 hospitalized patients with CDI to 38,644 hospitalized patients without CDI during the calendar year of 2009. They found that 13% of the CDI patients compared with 2.7% of the non-CDI patients died during their hospital stay. After adjustment for age, gender and co-morbidity, the relative risk of pre-discharge death for patients with CDI was 2.74%, and the proportion of hospital deaths due to CDI was 1.72%.

Psychological impact of acquiring CDI

There appears to be no recent research on the psychological impact of CDI, but it would be prudent to think that Pegues' (2013) concerns regarding MRSA will be mirrored for CDI.

Financial impact of CDI

Hospital acquired CDI significantly prolongs a patient's length of stay in hospital and therefore the cost of caring for that patient (Forster et al. 2010).

It must be noted, however, that their study does not include a formal cost analysis. Lipp et al. (2012) in their research examining the impact of hospital acquired CDI in New York State, from 2007 to 2008, analysed 4,853,800 patient discharges and found an incidence rate of 0.8 cases per 1000 discharged patients. They estimated that this accounted for 23,000 additional bed days amounting to an annual cost of approximately $55 million. This is a major burden to the US health system.

Activity

- Have you worked in a healthcare facility where either MRSA or CDI was diagnosed?
- How many patients were infected?
- How did your organization deal with the infection?
- Was this appropriate?

Ventilator-acquired pneumonia (VAP)

Nosocomial infections are common complications of a hospital stay (Burke 2003). Of these, ventilator-acquired pneumonia (VAP) represents 5%–18% of all infections (Shorr and Kollef 2005).

VAP is a common hazardous complication in mechanically ventilated patients and is associated with increased morbidity and mortality in critically ill patients (Sinuff et al. 2013). VAP is defined as pneumonia that occurs in mechanically ventilated patients more than 48 to 72 hours after endotracheal intubation (Gu et al. 2012). Early-onset VAP occurs 48 to 96 hours after intubation, and late-onset VAP is usually seen 96 hours after intubation (Augustyn 2007).

VAP is the most common infection seen in ICUs and accounts for one-fourth of the infections occurring in critically ill patients and half the antibiotic prescriptions in mechanically ventilated patients. In addition to being a financial burden in ICUs due to increased length of stay and associated costs, it continues to contribute significantly to the morbidity and mortality of ICU patients, with an estimated attributable mortality rate of 8%–15% (Ashraf and Ostrosky-Zeichner 2012).

The incidence of VAP varies between 9% and 27% in Europe and the USA (Rea-Neto et al. 2008) and rises to 41% in low-income countries (Rosenthal et al. 2006). Data from the United States National Nosocomial Infection Surveillance (NNIS) system showed that 31% of nosocomial infections were nosocomial pneumonia (Richards et al. 1999). Of those, 95% were associated with the use of mechanical ventilation. VAP is attributable to 20% to 50% of deaths in patients on mechanical ventilation; the mortality rate can be up to 70% in patients with multi-resistant infections (Rea-Neto et al. 2008). One study reported that the mortality rate of patients with VAP is twice as high as patients without VAP (Safdar et al. 2005).

There are no current data on the incidence of VAP in the UK; however, data from the USA suggests that it affects 9–27% of all intubated patients with approximately five cases per 1000 ventilator days (Hunter 2012). In 2011 the Department of Health published a High Impact Intervention Care Bundle to reduce the incidence of VAP and NICE guidelines were drawn up to support this. They are now used nationwide for all ventilated patients and considered as standardization of best practice in the management of a ventilated patient.

According to the Department of Health (2011), VAP is the most frequent infection occurring in patients after admission to the ICU (Vincent et al. 2006). In a recent large European observational study, almost 25% of patients developed an ICU-acquired infection, and the respiratory site accounted for 80% of these infections. The attributable mortality of VAP continues to be debated (Melson et al. 2009), but VAP can be linked with increased duration of ventilation, ICU and hospital length of stay, and significantly increased costs (Safdar et al. 2005). Prevention of VAP is possibly one of the most cost-effective interventions currently attainable in the ICU (Shorr and Wunderink 2003).

However, despite the implementation of the VAP care bundle and its supporting literature, the incidence of VAP remains high.

Financial impact of VAP

As stated above, VAP increases LOS and as a result significantly increases financial costs. Kollef et al. (2012), in their retrospective matched cohort study found that, of 87,689 patients admitted to ICUs and receiving ventilation for more than two days, 2.5% had VAP and the incidence rate was 1.27 per 1000 ventilation days. Patients with VAP had longer mechanical ventilation days (21.8 versus 10.3), a longer ICU stay (20.5 versus 11.6 days) and a longer hospitalization period (32.6 versus 19.5 days) than patients without VAP. Hospitalization costs for patients with VAP was US$99,598 compared with US$59,770, or a difference of US$39,828.

Violence, bullying and aggression (VBA)

The Health and Safety Executive (HSE) defines workplace violence as 'Any incident in which a person is abused, threatened or assaulted in circumstances relating to their work' (Health and Safety Executive 2013).

Healthcare workers encounter physical assaults and non-physical violence across the globe (in China, Wu et al. 2012; in the USA, Hartley et al. 2012; in Turkey, Ayranci et al. 2006; in Thailand, Kamchuchat et al. 2008; in Australia, Cashmore et al. 2012; in South Africa, Kennedy and Page 2012). Violence can take many forms, including physical assault, threats of physical violence, unwanted sexual advances and harassment. In nursing, patients, the families of patients, visitors or colleagues can commit violence, and nurses working in inpatient psychiatric facilities, nursing homes and emergency departments are thought to be the most at risk (Roche et al. 2010). Additionally, horizontal violence (nurse against nurse) is well documented and has been shown to affect the quality and safety of patient care (Purpora and Blegen 2012). Walrafen et al. (2012) list nine negative behaviours associated with horizontal violence:

- non-verbal negative innuendo (e.g. face-making, raising eyebrow)
- covert or overt verbal affront (e.g. withholding information, abrupt responses)
- undermining clinical activities (turning away when asked for help)
- sabotage (deliberately setting up a negative situation)
- bickering among peers
- scapegoating (e.g. assigning blame)
- backstabbing
- failure to respect the privacy of others (e.g. gossiping)
- broken commitments or broken confidences.

Most healthcare workers do not report violent incidents, due, in part, to the fact that they see violence as 'part of the territory' (Kennedy and Page 2012). However, the physical and psychological impact of violence, at whatever level, can result in higher absenteeism, increased turnover, decreased job satisfaction and lower productivity.

Spector et al. (2014) in their systematic review of 136 articles, reported five types of violence:

1. Physical
2. Non-physical
3. Bullying
4. Sexual harassment
5. Combined (type of violence was not indicated).

The overall exposure rates were

- physical violence: 36.4%
- non-physical: 66.9%
- bullying: 39.7%
- sexual harassment: 25%
- nurses having been physically injured in an assault: 32.7%.

Physical violence was most prevalent in emergency departments, geriatric, and psychiatric facilities. Physical violence and sexual harassment were most prevalent in Anglo countries, and non-physical violence and bullying were most prevalent in the Middle East. Patients were the perpetrators of most physical violence in Anglo countries and Europe, and patients' families and friends accounted for the most in the Middle East.

Hutchinson et al. (2013), in their editorial in the *Journal of Clinical Nursing*, discuss what has been learnt in five years of scholarship on VBA. Drawing on a number of articles that have been published in the *Journal of Clinical Nursing* since 2008, they present a summary of international research in this area:

- Many nurses encounter VBA in their workplaces.
- VBA has an impact on both nurses and workplace relationships and practices.
- VBA is often gendered and sexualized.
- Repeated VBA damages personal well-being, motivation, work performance, job satisfaction, social and personal identity.
- Violence remains under-reported despite reporting processes.
- In some setting, policy is under-developed.
- VBA seems to occur in an environment of passive agreement, that is, others are present when it takes place.
- VBA, as well as impacting the individual, has a significant impact on workplace culture, workplace behaviour and workplace leadership.
- Although not stated in the literature, it is stated anecdotally that bullying often takes place in front of patients and this may have an impact on patients, carers and patient care.

Activity

- Have you been the victim of VBA?
- What systems are in place in your workplace to reduce this?
- What else can be done to reduce the incidence of VBA where you work?

Pressure ulcers (PUs)

Pressure ulcers (PUs) are a common but usually preventable condition most often seen in older adults. PUs often develop over bony prominences, and incidence rates vary by clinical setting; for example, 0.4%–38% in acute care, 2.2%–23.9% in long-term care and 0%–17% in home care (Holroyd-Leduc and Reddy 2012). PUs are generally a marker of poor overall prognosis and may, due to sepsis, contribute to mortality.

However, PUs can also occur in children, and in particular those related to medical device-related (MDR) hospital acquired pressure ulcers (HAPUs). Paediatric MDR HAPUs are increasing, and their management and emotional suffering have a great impact on the health status of infants and children (Murray et al. 2013). This is supported by Boesch et al. (2012), whose work centred on the reduction of tracheostomy-related pressure ulcers (TRPUs). They found that the introduction of a quality improvement programme using a rapid-cycle Plan-Do-Study-Act (PDSA) framework resulting in the implementation of a clinical bundle significantly reduced the incidence of TRPUs in their ventilator unit.

A further quality improvement (QI) project was undertaken by Visscher et al. (2013), who aimed to reduce PUs in their ICUs by 50%. Their study included 1425 patients over 54,351 patient stays in the Paediatric Intensive Care Unit (PICU) and Neonatal Intensive Care Unit (NICU). They initiated a QI leadership team, measured PU rates, developed a QI bundle and audited the PU rates after implementation. They achieved a 50% reduction in PUs in the PICU, but no significant reduction in the NICU.

Psychological impact of PUs

Researchers have recently shown an interest in the psychological impact of PUs. Gorecki et al. (2009) conducted a systematic review in which they reviewed the responses of 2463 adults with PUs in hospitals, the community and long-term care settings. Their research spanned Europe, the Unites States, Asia and Australia. They found that PUs had a significant impact on patients and their families and quality of life. The research also highlighted what patients see as social isolation, as they are concerned about what others will think about wound leakage and smell.

Financial impact of PUs

PUs result in longer LOS, and treatment is costly. The cost of treating PUs in the UK in 2004 was thought to be £1.4 to £2.1 billion (Bennett et al. 2004). An estimated $11 billion is spent every year in the USA (Holroyd-Leduc and Reddy 2012).

PUs are a financial drain in the UK and impact both on patients and healthcare providers (Dealey et al. 2012). Using August 2011 prices, Dealey et al. investigated the cost of treating PUs by looking at the daily resource allocation required to deliver good clinical practice. They estimated that the cost of treating a category one PU was £1214 and £14,108 for treating a category five PU. The higher cost was related to the length of time needed to heal the ulcer and the additional complications found with more severe cases.

Activity

- Have you treated a patient with a PU?
- Find the articles by Boesch et al. (2012) and Visscher et al. (2013) to see how you might lead a quality improvement project to reduce the incidence of PUs in your workplace.

Medication errors

Whilst many medication errors cause little or no harm, some can cause great harm, and all are preventable (Agrawal et al. 2009). Medication errors occur in all settings and at all levels of care.

Avery et al. (2012) published a piece of work looking at medication errors in general practice. The study looked at 6048 prescription items for 1777 patients. Errors were found in 1 in 8 patients or approximately 1 in 20 prescriptions. Most errors were mild to moderate but 550 items demonstrated severe error and errors were not associated with the experience of the GP. The conclusion of the study was that medication errors in general practices are common, but severe errors are unusual.

In paramedic emergency care, the scope for medication error increases as the scope for paramedic practice increases (Crossman 2009). Crossman (2009) suggests that, whilst there has been much research on medication error in primary, secondary and community care, little attention has been focused on the prehospital environment. The prehospital environment is sometimes unpredictable and uncontrolled. Paramedics may be required to work in an environment where the possibility of medication error is increased, and delivering the highest level of care in adverse environments such as

- danger and possible abuse from patient, relatives, bystanders
- limited light or darkness
- adverse weather conditions
- distractions from noise, traffic, bystanders
- cramped or moving work environment
- remote settings
- inability to gain essential information such as medical history, medication history and medication allergies from the patient.

Such settings may make it difficult for the paramedic to follow McGovern's (1992) golden rules:

- Administer the right drug.
- Administer the drug to the right patient.
- Administer the right dose.
- Administer the drug by the right route.
- Administer the drug at the right time.
- Teach the patient about the drugs they have been given.
- Take a complete patient drug history.
- Consider potential drug interactions.
- Document each drug administered.

Furthermore, the consequences of medication error by paramedics may be compounded by the difficulty of identifying prehospital care errors, and errors not identified by the paramedic are likely to be unnoticed, for example an overly high dose of nitroglycerin in a prehospital setting might result in a hospital diagnosis of cardiac failure, rather than drug overdose (Hobgood et al. 2006). Interestingly, in a study undertaken by Lifschitz et al. (2011) in Israel, more medication errors occurred in the Emergency Department than in emergency vehicles.

In secondary care, Kelly et al. (2011), in their observational study of 65 drug rounds on care-of-older persons wards, found that, of the 2129 drug administrations to 625 patients, 817 doses (38.4%) were given incorrectly.

Desai et al. (2013) carried out a cross-sectional analysis of medication error incidents in nursing homes in North Carolina between 2010 and 2011 and found that 32,176 individual medication errors were reported to the Medication Error Quality Initiative during this period. The ten classes of drugs most commonly associated with medication errors were

1. Analgesics (12.27%)
2. Anxiolytics/sedatives/hypnotics (8.39%)
3. Antidiabetic agents (5.86%)
4. Anticoagulants (5.04%)
5. Anticonvulsants (4.05%)
6. Andidepressants (4.05%)
7. Laxatives (3.13%)
8. Ophthalmic preparations (2.77%)
9. Antipsychotics (2.47%)
10. Diuretics (2.34%).

The correlation between usage and incidence of errors was not significant, suggesting that certain classes of drugs were more likely to be involved in medication errors regardless of the extent of their use.

Falls in the elderly

People are living longer and falls are a leading cause of injury and death in the elderly (Huang et al. 2012) thus falls are considered a major public health issue in older people (Palvanen et al. 2013). This group of patients falls for a number of reasons, including the following:

- changes in physical function and physiology
- the use (and misuse) of medications to manage polymorbidity.

Falls in the elderly living in the community

Ganz et al. (2007) in their systematic review of falls in patients aged 65 and over and living in the community found that

- the probability of a person over 65 falling once a year was 27%
- patients who have fallen once are likely to fall again.

The predictors of future falls were

- abnormalities in gait and balance
- visual impairment
- medication
- decreased activities of daily living
- impaired cognition.

Tung (2012) stated that, worldwide, falls are the second leading cause of accidental death and adults over the age of 65 are most prone to fatal falls. Additionally, non-fatal falls result in an adverse effect on quality of life due to soft tissue injuries, fractures (such as fractures to the proximal humerus, distal forearm, vertebrae, pelvis, hip and tibial condyles), dislocation or chronic pain (Karisson et al. 2013). Karisson et al. found that physical exercise, including balance and strength training, was the only intervention that reduced the number of falls and the number of fallers living in the community. Home hazard alterations, led by occupational therapists, reduced falls in the elderly living at home. A variety of modifications also seemed to reduce falls:

- Vitamin D supplement in those with low levels of Vitamin D
- modification of multipharmacy
- modification of psychotropic medication
- anti-slip shoes
- podiatry for patients with foot disability
- cataract surgery and pacemakers for patients with cardio-inhibitor carotid sinus hypersensitivity are surgical procedures that can reduce the risk of falls.

Falls in hospitalized elderly

According to Neumann et al. (2013), falls in the hospitalized elderly are frequent. The participants in their study were 4735 patients over the age of 65, and in this group, 10.7% had a fall with a fall rate of 7.9/1000 hospital days. Altered mental state, previous fall history and poor mobility had the strongest association to falls.

Psychological impact of a fall

Collerton et al. (2012) found that patients in their study reported a loss of confidence after a fall (40%), leaving the house less often (25.9%) and a worry about falling again (42%). All of the above were reported more by women than men.

Financial impact of falls in the elderly

Life expectancy, in the USA, has increased from 75 years in 1990 to 79 years in 2009, and it has been estimated that the number of people over 65 will double by 2050 (Boye et al. 2013). During 2000, falls accounted for close to 750,000 admissions and 45% of all inpatient injury related admissions. Fractures were the most common diagnosis, with 314,006 hip fractures. In the USA, in 2006, fall related costs were US$19 billion with an additional US$0.2 billion for fatal injuries.

Collerton et al. (2012) focused their study on the over 85s, the fastest growing age group in the UK. They found that of the participants who had fallen in the previous 12 months, 30.1% attended AandE, 12.8% were admitted and 10.6% had a fracture. And 4.5% attended AandE again and 1.9% were admitted more than once for the same incident. Patients living in a care home were more likely to fracture and require hospital admission than those living in their own homes.

They estimated that the average 12 month cost to the NHS per faller was £202 when applied to all the participants in the study (fallers and non-fallers), with the average cost of a single fall being £109, £65 of which relates to AandE services.

In-hospital falls are also common and have a financial impact. Coussement et al. (2008) reported that 2–12% of admissions result in a fall, while Krauss et al. (2007) found that falls cause harm in up to 40% of inpatients.

Application to your practice

Activity
Reflect on your own area of practice: • What are the possible quality issues in your area of practice? • What is the incidence, morbidity and mortality of these issues? • How have you been involved with these issues? • What was your role if you were involved?

Key point summary

In this chapter, seven incidents (NSIs, HAIs, VAP, VBA, pressure ulcers, medication errors and falls in the older population) have been discussed, demonstrating incidence, morbidity, mortality, psychological impact and financial impact on the organization. The fact that these issues still occur in a climate of clinical governance illustrates that we are not yet fully mindful of and responsible for the tenets of clinical governance.

- All staff regardless of grade should follow standard precautions and report all NSIs.
- Staff need to be mindful of the risks of acquiring incurable diseases through NSIs, for example Hepatitis C and HIV.
- Acquiring these diseases can impact significantly on staff and their families.
- HAIs, for example MRSA and *Clostridium difficile*, are potentially lethal and can have a significant financial impact on the organization.
- VAP is the most common infection on ICUs, accounting for one fourth of the infections occurring in critically ill patients and has a significant financial impact on the organization (due to increased length of stay).
- Staff working in emergency departments, geriatric and psychiatric facilities are most at risk of VBA, and the incidence is under-reported.
- Pressure ulcers can occur in all patients and are usually preventable. Lack of resources, for example insufficient staff and lack of specialist equipment, and poor guidelines, contribute to this largely avoidable condition.
- Whilst many medication errors cause little or no harm, a minority can cause great harm and all are preventable.
- Falls are a leading cause of injury and death in the older population in all healthcare settings. This will become an increasing problem as demographics change.

Implications for practice

- It is important to make sure you are cognisant of all policies relating to all these incidents.
- Always report 'near misses' and actual events and attend Occupational Health as necessary.
- Be mindful of not only the physical impact but also the psychological and financial repercussions of these issues.

End-of-chapter questions

- Does your place of work have clear policies pertaining to all of these issues? Do you know where to find them? Are they written in a language that is useful and meaningful to you?
- Which aspects of the clinical governance framework can best be applied to assist with a reduction of incidence?

See the Appendix on page 192 for suggested answers to these questions.

References

Agrawal A, Aronson JK, Britten N, Ferner RE, de Smet PA, Fialova D, Fitzgerald RJ, Likic R, Maxwell RE, Meyboom RH, Minuz P, Onder G, Schachter M, Velo G (2009) Medication errors: Problems and recommendations from a consensus meeting. *British Journal of Clinical Pharmacology*, 67, 592–598

Ashraf M and Ostrosky-Zeichner L (2012) Ventilator-associated pneumonia: A review. *Hospital Practice*, 40 (1), 93–105

Augustyn B. (2007) Ventilator-associated pneumonia: Risk factors and prevention. *Critical Care Nurse*, 27 (4), 32–39.

Avery AA, Barber N, Ghaleb M, Dean Franklin B, Armstrong S, Crowe S, Dhillon S, Freyer A, Howard R, Pezzoles C, Serumaga B, Swanwick G and Olanrewaju T (2012) *Investigating the prevalence and causes of prescribing errors in general practice: The PRACtICe Study*. Project Report. London: General Medical Council

Ayranci U, Yenilmex C, Balci Y and Keptanoglu C (2006) Identification of violence in Turkish healthcare settings. *Journal of interpersonal Violence*, 21 (2), 276–296

Badger VO, Ledeboer NA, Graham MB and Edmiston CE (2012) *Clostridium difficile*: Epidemiology, pathogenesis, management and prevention of a recalcitrant healthcare-associated pathogen. *Journal of Parenteral and Enteral Nutrition*, 36 (6), 645–662

Bennett G, Dealey C and Posnett D (2004) The cost of pressure ulcers in the UK. *Age and Ageing*, 33 (3), 230–235

Best EL, Fawley WN, Parnell P and Wilcox MH (2010) The potential for airborne dispersal of *Clostridium difficile* from symptomatic patients. *Clinical Infectious Diseases*, 50 (11), 1450–1457

Boesch PR, Myers C, Garrett R, Nie AM, Thomas N, Chima A, McPhail GL, Edmick M, Rutter MT and Dressman K (2012) Prevention of tracheostomy-related pressure ulcers in children. *Pediatrics*, 129 (3), 792–797

Boye NDA, Van Lieshout EMM, Van Beeck EF, Hartolt KA, Van der Camme TSM and Patka P (2013) The impact of falls in the elderly. *Trauma*, 13 (1), 29–35

Burke JP (2003) Infection control – a problem for patient safety. *New England Journal of Medicine*, 348, 651–656

Cashmore AW, Indig D, Hampton SE, Hegney DG, Jalaludin BB (2012) Workplace violence in a large correctional health service in New South Wales, Australia: A retrospective review of incident management reports. *BMC Health Services Research*, 12, 245–254

Collerton J, Kingston A, Davies K, Eccles MP, Jagger C, Kirkwood TB and Newton JL (2012) The personal and health service impact of falls in 85 year olds: Cross-sectional findings form the Newcastle 85+ Cohort Study. Available at http://www.plosone.org/article/info%3Adoi%2F10.1371%2Fjournal.pone.0033078 (accessed 15.8.13)

Coussement J, De Paepe L, Schwendimann R, Denhaerynck K, Dejaeger E, Milisen K (2008) Interventions for preventing falls in acute- and chronic-care hospitals: A systematic review and meta-analysis. *Journal of the American Geriatric Society*, 56 (1), 29–36

Crossman M (2009) Technical and environmental impact on paramedic practice: A review of causes, consequences and strategies for prevention. *Journal of Emergency Primary Healthcare*, 7 (3). Available at http://ro.ecu.edu.au/jephc/vol7/iss3/4 (accessed 28.1.14)

D'Agata EM, Webb GE, Horn MA, Moellering RC and Ruan S (2009) Modeling the invasion of community-acquired methicillin-resistant *Staphylococcus aureus* into hospitals. *Clinical Infectious Diseases*, 48, 274–284

Dealey C, Posnett J and Walker A (2012) The cost of pressure ulcers in the United Kingdom. *Journal of Wound Care*, 21 (6), 261–266

Department of Health (2007) High impact intervention: Care bundle to reduce the risk from *Clostridium difficile*. Available at http://hcai.dh.gov.uk/files/2011/03/Document_Clostridium_difficile_Infection_High_Impact_Intervention_FINAL_101210.pdf (accessed 25.3.13)

Department of Health (2011) High impact intervention to reduce ventilator associated Pneumonia. Available at http://webarchive.nationalarchives.gov.uk/20120118164404/hcai.dh.gov.uk/files/2011/03/2011-03-14-HII-Ventilator-Associated-Pneumonia-FINAL.pdf (accessed 08.02.13)

Desai RJ, Williams CE, Greene SB, Pierson S, Caprio AJ and Hansen RA (2013) Exploratory evaluation of medication classes most commonly involved in nursing home errors. *Journal of the American Directors Association*, 14, 6, 403–408

Directive 2010/32/EU Prevention from sharp injuries in the hospital and healthcare sector. Available at https://www.osha.europa.eu/en/legislation/directives/sector-specific-and-worker-related-provisions/osh-dirctives/council-directive-2010-32-eu (accessed 30.03.2013)

Elder A and Paterson C (2006) Sharps injuries in UK healthcare: A review of injury rates, viral transmission and potential efficacy of safety devices. *Occupational Medicine*, 56, 566–574

Elmiyeh B, Whitaker IS, James MJ, Chahal CAA, Galea A and Alshafi K (2004) Needlestick injuries in the National Health Service: A culture of silence. *Journal of the Royal Society of Medicine*, 97 (7), 326–327

Enoch DA and Aliyu SH (2012) Is *Clostridium difficile* infection still a problem for hospitals? *Canadian Medical Association Journal*, 184, 17–18

Enright MC, Robinson DA, Randle G, Feil EJ, Grundmann H and Spratt BG (2002) The evolutionary history of methicillin-resistant *Staphylococcus aureas* (MRSA). *Proceedings of the National Academy of Sciences*, 99 (11) 7687–7692

Forster AJ, Taljaard M, Oake N, Wilson K, Roth V and van Walraven C (2010) The effect of hospital-acquired infection with *Clostridium difficile* on length of stay in hospital. *Canadian Medical Association Journal*, 184, 37–42

Ganz DA, Bao Y, Shekelle PG and Rubenstein LZ (2007) Will my patient fall? *Journal of the American Medical Association*, 297 (1), 77–86

Gershon RRM, Quereshi KA, Pogorzelska M, Rosen J, Gebbie KM, Brandt-Rauf PW and Sherman ME (2007) Non-hospital based registered nurses and the risk of blood born pathogen exposure. *Industrial Health*, 45 (5), 697–704

Gorecki C, Brown JM, Nelson EA, Briggs M, Schoonhoven L, Dealey C, Defloor T, Nixon J (European Quality of Life Pressure Ulcer Project group) (2009) Impact of pressure ulcers on quality of life in older patients: A systematic review. *Journal American Geriatric Society*, 57 (7), 1175–1183

Gosbell DB (2004) Methicillin-resistant *Staphylococcus aureus*. *American Journal of Clinical Dermatology*, 5 (4), 239–259

Green B and Griffiths EC (2103) Psychiatric consequences of needle stick injury. *Occupational Medicine Advance Access*. Available at http://occmed.oxfordjournals.org/content/early/2013/02/20/occmed.kqt006.full.pdf.html (accessed 25.3.13)

Gu W-J, Gong Y-Z, Lei P, No Yu-Xia, Liu J-C (2012) Impact of oral care with versus without toothbrushing on the prevention of ventilator-associated pneumonia: A systematic review and meta-analysis of randomized controlled trials. *Critical Care*, 16 (R190), 2–9

Hardy K, Manzoor S, Marriott C, Parsons H, Waddlington C, Gossain S, Szczepura A, Stallard N and Hawkey PM (2012) Utilizing rapid multiple-locus variable-number tandem-repeat analysis typing to aid control of hospital-acquired *Clostridium difficile* infection: A multicenter study. *Journal of Clinical Microbiology*, 50 (10), 3244–3248

Hartley D, Doman B, Hendricks SA, Jenkins EL (2012) Non-fatal workplace violence injuries in the United States 2003–2004: A follow back study. *Work: A Journal of Prevention, Assessment and Rehabilitation*, 42 (1), 125–135

Health and Safety Executive, *Work-related Violence*. Available at http://www.hse.gov.uk/violence (accessed 11.07.13)

Health Protection Agency Centre for Infections, National Public Health Service for Wales, CDSC Northern Ireland and Health Protection Scotland (2008) *Eye of the needle: surveillance of significant occupational exposure to blood borne viruses in healthcare workers*. London: HPA

Hiko D, Jemal A, Sudhakar M, Kerie MW, Dejene T (2012) Effectiveness of training on standard precautions to prevent needle stick injuries among health professionals: A systematic review. *JBI Database of Systematic Reviews*, 10 (14), 201–213

Hobgood C, Bowen JB, Brice JH, Overby B, Tamayo-Sarver JH (2006) Do EMS personel identify, report and disclose medical errors? *Prehospital Emergency Care*, 10 (1), 80–84

Holroyd-Leduc Y and Reddy M (2012) *Evidence based geriatric medicine: a practical clinical guide*. Oxford: Wiley-Blackwell

Huang AR, Mallet L, Rochefort CM, Eguale T, Buckeridge D and Tamblyn R (2012) Medication-related falls in the elderly: Causative factors and preventive strategies. *Drugs and Aging*, 29 (5), 359–376

Hudson LO, Murphy CR, Spratt BG, Enright MC, Terpstra L, Gombosev A, Hannah P, Mikhail L, Alexander R, Moore D and Huang S (2011) Differences in methicillin-resistant *Staphylococcus aureus* isolated from pediatric and adult patients from hospital in a large county in California. *Journal of Clinical Microbiology*, 50 (3), 573–579

Hunter J (2012) Ventilator associated pneumonia. *British Medical Journal*. Available at http://www.bmj.com/content/344/bmj.e3325 (accessed 08.02.13)

Hutchinson M, Jackson D, Haigh C, Hayter M (2013) Editorial: five years of scholarship on violence, bullying and aggression towards nurses in the workplace: What have we learned? *Journal of Clinical Nursing*, 22, 903–905

Joint WHO/ILO Guidelines on health services and HV/AIDS (2005). Available at www.who.int/hiv/pub/guidelines/ilowhoguidelines_ru.pdf (accessed 12.8.13)

Kamchuchat C, Chongsuvivatwong V, Oncheunjit S, Yip TM, Sangthong (2008) Workplace violence directed at nursing staff at a general hospital in Southern Thailand (2008) *Journal of Occupational Health*, 55 (2), 201–207

Karisson ME, Vonschewelov T, Karisson C, Coster M and Rosengen B (2013) Prevention of falls in the elderly: A review. *Scandinavian Journal of Public Health*, 41 (5), 442–454

Kelly J, Wright D and Wood J (2011) Medicine administration errors in patients with dysphagia in secondary care: a multi-centre observational study. *Journal of Advanced Nursing*, 67 (12), 2615–2627

Kennedy M and Page JH (2012) Nurses' experiences and understating of workplace violence in a trauma and emergency department in South Africa. *Health SA Gesondheid*, 18 (1), 1–11

Klein SL, Kowalski CP, Hofer TP and Saint S (2011) Preventing hospital acquired infections: A national survey of practices reported by U.S. Hospitals in 2005 and 2009. Available at http://link.springer.com/article/10.1007%2Fs11606-011-1935-y?LI=truepage-1 (accessed 25.3.13)

Kollef MH, Hamilton CW and Ernst F (2012) Economic impact of ventilator-associated pneumonia in a large matched cohort. *Infection Control and Hospital Epidemiology*, 33 (3), 250–256

Krauss MJ, Nguyen SL and Dunagan WC (2007) Circumstances of patient falls and injuries in nine hospitals in a Midwestern health-care system. *Infection Control and Hospital Epidemiology*, 28 (5), 544–550

Leigh JP, Wiatrowski WJ, Gillen M, Steenland NK (2008) Characteristics of persons and jobs with needle stick injury in a national data set. *American Journal of Infection Control*, 36, 414–420

Lifshitz AE, Goldstein LH, Sharist M, Strugo R, Assulin E, BarHaim S, Feigenberg Z, Berkovitch M and Kozer E (2012) Medication prescribing errors in the pre hospital setting and in the ED *American Journal of Emergency Medicine*, 30 (5), 726–731

Lipp MJ, Nero DC and Callahan MA (2012) Impact of hospital-acquired *Clostridium difficile*. *Journal of Gastroenterology and Hepatology*, 27 (11), 1733–1737

Macedo-Vinas M, De Angelis G, Rohner P, Safran E, Stewardson A, Franhauser C, Schrenzel J, Pittet D and Harbarth S (2013) Burden of methicillin-resistant *Staphylococcus aureus* infections at a Swiss University Hospital: Excess length of stay and costs. *Journal of Hospital Medicine*, 84 (2), 132–137

McGovern K (1992) Ten golden rules for administering drugs safely. *Nursing*, 22 (3), 49–56

Melson WG, Rovers MM and Bonten MJM (2009) Ventilator-associated pneumonia and mortality: A systematic review of observational studies. *Critical Care Medicine*, 39, 2709–2718

Murray JRD (2009) The incidence and reporting rates of needle stick injury among UK surgeons. *Annals of the Royal College of Surgeons of England*, 91 (1), 12–17

Murray JS, Noonan C, Quigley S and Curley M (2013) Medical device-related hospital-acquired pressure ulcers in children: An integrative review. *Journal of Paediatric Nursing*, 28 (6), 585–595

Naghavi SHR, Shabestari O and Alcolado J (2013) Post-traumatic stress disorder in trainee doctors with previous needle stick injury. *Occupational Medicine (London)*, 63 (4), 247

Neumann L, Hoffman VS, Golgert S, Hasford A and von Rentein-Kruise W (2013) In-hospital fall-risk screening in 4,735 geriatric patients for the LUCAS project. *Journal of Nutrition, Health and Aging*, 17 (3), 264–269

Palaven M, Kannus P, Piirtola M, Miemi S, Parkkan S and Jarvinen M (2013) Effectiveness of the Chaos Falls Clinic in preventing falls and injuries in home-dwelling older adults: A randomized controlled trial. Available at http://www.sciencedirect.com/science/articles/pii/S0020138313001332 (accessed 14.8.13)

Papenburg J, Blais D, Moore D, Al-Hosni M, Lafferiere C, Tapiero B and Quach C (2008) Pediatric injuries from needs discarded in the community: Epidemiology and risk of seroconversion. *Pediatrics*, 122 (2), 487–492

Pathak R, Kahlon KH, Ahluwalia SK, Sharma S, Bhardwaj R (2012) Needle stick injury and inadequate post exposure practices among healthcare workers in a tertiary care centre in rural India. *International Journal of Collaborative Research on Internal Medicine and Public Health*, 4 (5), 638

Pegues DA (2013) How to maximize the benefit and reduce the unintended consequences of contract precautions for control of methicillin-resistant *Staphilococcus aureus*. *Clinical Infectious Diseases*, 57 (20), 185–187

Popovich KJ, Hota B, Aroutcheva A, Kurien L, Patel J, Lyles-Banks R, Grasso AE, Spec A, Beavis KG, Hayden MK and Weinstein RA (2013) Community-associated methicillin-resistant *Staphyloccocus aureus* burden in HIV-infected patients. *Journals of the Royal Society of Tropical Medicine and Hygiene*, 56 (8), 1067–1074

Purpora C and Blegen MA (2012) Horizontal violence and the quality and safety of patient care: a conceptual model. *Nursing Practice and Research*. Available at http://www.dx.doi.org/10.1155/2012/306948 (accessed 24.1.14)

Rea-Neto A, Youssef NC, Tuche F, Brunkhorst F, Ranieri VM, Reinhart K (2008) Diagnosis of ventilator-associated pneumonia: A systematic review of the literature. *Critical Care*, 12 (2), R56 (doi:10.1186/cc6877).

Richards MJ, Edwards JR, Culver DH, Gaynes RP (1999) Nosocomial infections in medical intensive care units in the United States: National Nosocomial Infections Surveillance System. *Critical Care Medicine*, 27 (8), 887–892

Roche M, Diers D, Duffield C and Catling-Paull C (2010) Violence toward nurses, the work environment and patient outcomes. *Journal of Nursing Scholarship*, 42 (1), 13–22

Rosenthal VD, Maki DG, Salomao R, Moreno CA, Mehta Y, Higuera F (2006) Device-associated nosocomial infections in 55 intensive care units of eight developing countries. *Annals of Internal Medicine*, 145 (8), 582–591

Safdar N, Dezfulian C, Collard HR, Saint S (2005) Clinical and economic consequences of ventilator-associated pneumonia: A systematic review. *Critical Care Medicine*, 33, 2184–2193

Scaggiante R, Chemello L, Rinaldi R, Bartolucci GV and Trevisan A (2013) Acute hepatitis C infection in a nurse trainee following a needle stick injury. *World Journal of Gastroenterology*, 19 (4), 501–505

Sharma A, Gur R and Bhalia P (2012) Study on the prevalence of needle stick injury among healthcare workers in a tertiary care hospital in New Delhi: A two-year review. *Indian Journal of Public Health*, 56, 101–103

Shorr AF and Kollef MH (2005) Ventilator-associated pneumonia: Insights from recent clinical trials. *Chest Journal*, 128 (Suppl 2), 583–591

Shorr AF and Wunderink RG (2003) Dollars and sense in the intensive care unit: The costs of ventilator associated pneumonia. *Critical Care Medicine*, 31, 1582–1583

Sinuff T, Muscedere J, Cook DJ, Dodek PM, Anderson W, Keenan SP, Wood G, Tan R, Haupt MT, Miletin M, Bouali R, Jiang X, Day AG, Overvelde J, Heyland DK (2013) Implementation of clinical practice guidelines for ventilator-associated pneumonia: A multicentre prospective study. *Critical Care Medicine*, 41 (1), 15–23

Sohn J-W, Kim B-G, Kim S-H and Han C (2006) Mental health of healthcare workers who experience needle stick and sharps injuries. *Journal of Occupational Health*, 48, 474–479

Song X, Bartlett JG, Speck KA, Naegeli A, Carroll K and Perl TM (2008) Rising economic impact of *Clostridium difficile*-associated disease in adult hospitalized patient population. *Infection Control and Hospital Epidemiology*, 29, 823–828

Spector PE, Zhou ZE and Che XX (2014) Nurse exposure to physical and nonphysical violence, bullying and sexual harassment: A quantitative review. *International Journal of Nursing Studies*, 51 (1), 72–84

Thomas WJC and Murray JRD (2009) The incidence and reporting rates of needle stick injury among UK surgeons. *Annals of the Royal College of Surgeons of England*, 91 (1), 12–17

Trueman P, Taylor M, Twena N and Chubb B (2008) The cost of needle stick injuries associated with insulin administration. *British Journal of Community Nursing*, 13, 413–417

Tung KK (2012) The effectiveness of virtual reality exercises for improving balance control, reducing fall risk and incidence among the frail elderly with a history of falls. Available at http://www.theses.lib.polyu.edu.hk (accessed 14.8.13)

Vincent J-L, Sakr Y, Sprung CD, Ranieri VM, Reinhart K, Gerlach H, Moreno R, Carlet J, Le Gall J-R, Payen D (2006) Sepsis in European intensive care units: Results of the SOAP study. *Critical Care Medicine*, 34 (2), 344–353

Visscher M, King A, Nie AP, Schaffer P, Taylor T, Pruitt D, Giaccone MJ, Ashby M and Keswani Sundeep (2013) *Pediatrics*, 131 (6), 1950–1960

Wada K, Sakata Y, Fujino Y (2007) The association of needle stick injury with depressive symptoms among first year medical residents in Japan. *Industrial Health*, 45, 750–755

Wallin TR, Hern GH and Frazee BW (2008) Community-associated methicillin-resistant *Staphylococcus aureus*. *Emergency Medicine Clinics of North America*, 26, 431–455

Walrafen N, Brewer MK and Mulvenon C (2012) Sadly caught up in the moment: An exploration of horizontal violence. *Nursing Economics*, 30 (1), 6–13

Wenisch JM, Schmid G, Tucek G, Kuo H-W, Allerberger F, Michi V, Tesik P, Laferi H and Wenisch C (2012) A prospective cohort study on hospital mortality due to *Clostridium difficile* infection. *Infection*, 40 (5), 479–484

WHO (2002) The world health report: Reducing risks, promoting health life. Geneva: WHO

Willburn SQ and Eijkemans G (2004) Preventing needle stick injuries among healthcare workers: a WHO-ICN collaboration. *International Journal of Occupational and Environmental Health*, 10, 451–456

Wu S, Lin S, Li H and Chai W (2012) A study of workplace violence and its effect on the quality of life among medical professionals in China. *Archives of Environmental and Occupational Health*, 69 (2), 81–88

3

Exploring quality failings within clinical contexts

Mary Gottwald

Chapter contents

- Learning objectives
- Introduction
- Quality circles
- Dimensions of quality: Maxwell 6
- Dimensions of quality: three organizational dimensions
- Ishikawa's fishbone
- SWOT
- PESTLE/PEST
- Key point summary
- Implications for practice
- End-of-chapter questions
- References

Learning objectives

By the end of this chapter, the reader will be better able to

- understand how quality circles can be used within quality management
- identify the dimensions of quality
- identify and use tools to analyse the causes of poor quality care
- compare and contrast a variety of analytical tools.

Introduction

The previous chapters have explored why the application of clinical governance is so important in today's practice and have discussed evidence linked to specific examples that highlight the incidence of poor quality healthcare. This chapter will begin by exploring how quality circles can be used to help health and social care teams initiate discussions around the quality of care provided. It will then explore and critique a number of tools that can be used to analyse the reasons why particular quality issues and poor standards of healthcare arise in practice. These tools will be applied to specific examples from practice.

There are a variety of tools and theories that can be used when defining quality and analysing the causes of quality issues in clinical governance. In this chapter we have chosen to focus on the following:

- Maxwell 6
- three organizational dimensions
- Ishikawa's fishbone
- SWOT
- PESTLE.

As discussed in chapter 1, it must be remembered that quality is a personal construct dependent on one's beliefs and values and therefore quality can be considered to link to one's perception. This presents a challenge to using any of these tools and we therefore need to be mindful of this.

Quality circles

Quality circles were established in Japan in 1962 and in the West in the 1970s (Ishikawa 1985). Although they originated within business, quality circles are a simple, well-used method that healthcare teams and service users can use to work together and begin discussions, for example to prioritize development of healthcare that is failing to meet required standards (such as those identified by NICE, discussed in chapter 1). These discussions provide an opportunity for managers, service users and healthcare professionals to share ideas, prioritize areas for improvement and agree the way forward using clinical governance strategies.

To establish a quality circle, there is a need for between three and twelve volunteers, working in the same practice area to form the circle. They need to have an interest in resolving specific issues within healthcare and need to agree to meet at frequent intervals to brainstorm appropriate issues (Mullins 2010, Moullin 2002, Sale 2005). Ishikawa (1985) places an emphasis on the 'volunteer' aspect, as this provides autonomy and empowerment for the members; he also suggests that teams should meet at a minimum twice a month, preferably weekly to begin with.

There are two key members that must be included in this group; the first is to have a manager, as they help practitioners to take their ideas forward. The second essential member is the inclusion of a patient, service user or relative, as they are the ones who have experience of the healthcare provided. Otherwise the members can include a range of professionals at different grades.

Key point

• Service users and managers are essential members of a quality circle.

Quality circles can be used both at the analysis stage and resolution stage and discussions in each of these stages will go through two phases:

1. Divergent phase
   a. General discussion on what the quality issues are.
   b. Prioritization of which quality issues to focus on.
   c. Analysis of causes that can be used to explain why the quality issue(s) has arisen.
   d. Identification of *all* potential ways to ameliorate problem(s).
2. Convergent phase
   a. Decision-making on which resolutions are feasible to implement.
   b. Decision-making on which clinical governance strategies can be used to resolve the quality issue and improve the patient experience.

Divergent phase

Firstly all members of the group will brainstorm the various quality issues and problems that have arisen, for example medication errors, falls in the older population, pressure sores, hospital acquired infections or workplace violence. To help with this discussion, it is useful for one member of the group to agree to record all suggestions either on a laptop or flip chart. Once all the issues have been identified, members discuss the quality issue(s) that can be resolved and prioritize which ones will be the main focus.

It is important to remember that not all problems are necessarily within the remit of the quality circle due to resource restraints. Also, if an issue that is reasonably easy to resolve is chosen initially, then this can promote motivation and enthusiasm with the group due to the potential successful resolution (Sale 2005).

Once the quality circle members have agreed on which quality issue to focus on, the group will begin the analysis. Using one of the tools that will be discussed below, the members of the group can brainstorm all the reasons that can be used to explain the causes of a specific quality issue.

The final stage of the divergent phase is for members to identify possible strategies and resolutions, and it is at this point that *all* suggestions are valued and noted. The divergent phase for implementing these strategies may include some quite heated debates, because as the group brainstorm all possible resolutions, some 'off the wall ideas' may be presented. These ideas, though, will often prompt other ideas, so can be useful.

Convergent phase

Following this brainstorming activity, the group will finally *converge* and identify the realistic ideas that can be operationalized. An action plan will need to be identified, and it is at this point that managers can help the team by taking the ideas forward.

Table 3.1 Critique of quality circles

Advantages	Disadvantages
• Easy to organize. • Promote the consultation process. • Promote collaboration between service users and practitioners. • Teams can become involved at the local level. • Motivate practitioners and service users. • Engage multidisciplinary practitioners and service users in problem-solving activities. • Promote understanding of different roles. • Provide autonomy for the members to select which problem to analyse and resolve. • Facilitate practitioners' understanding of quality processes. • Successful outcomes motivate and reward staff and service users. • Promote a strong organizational quality culture. • Minutes are taken and therefore show positive outcomes.	• Require planning. • Could be considered time consuming. • If not part of the formal structures, meetings may easily be cancelled due to workloads. • Without the support of managers, implementing the resolutions could be problematic. • De-motivating if the recommendations are not implemented. • De-motivating if there is resistance from senior staff. • Not part of the strategic planning level. • Cost implications if training is required; for example, for group facilitator, group leader, minute taker.

(Keleman 2005, Mullins 2010, Moullin 2002, Sale 2005)

There are a number of advantages and disadvantages to using this method for identifying quality issues. We have highlighted the main ones in table 3.1.

Activity

Reflect on your own area of practice:

• What would you need to do to organize a quality circle?
• How would you engage members to join the group?
• Which members would be appropriate?
• Does it matter who belongs to the quality circle?

Dimensions of quality: Maxwell 6

Two tools that demonstrate how quality can mean different things to different people are

1. Maxwell 6
2. Ovretveit's 3 Organizational Dimensions.

Maxwell argues that in order to be considered quality care, six dimensions need to be met. Whereas the focus of Ovretveit's model is on the relationship and conflict that could occur between three dimensions.

Maxwell 6

Maxwell (1984, 1992) argues that there are six dimensions that need to be considered when contextualizing quality:

1. Efficiency and economy
2. Effectiveness
3. Access
4. Social acceptability
5. Equity
6. Relevance.

These dimensions will help practitioners decide whether there is a problem with quality care or not. If there are issues with any of these dimensions, then Maxwell considers that a quality issue has arisen. Maxwell (1992:176) emphasizes that although these dimensions are a useful framework, they must not be taken 'too literally' and are therefore perhaps a starting point for practitioners to consider. Table 3.2 briefly explains what each of Maxwell's dimensions means.

Table 3.2 Dimensions of quality

Dimension	Care is not quality if . . .
Efficiency and economy	the intervention costs more than it needs to. So resources must not be misspent
Effectiveness	the evidence base has not been explored or implemented
Access	there are socioeconomic or geographical problems such as access to healthcare services and difficulties getting there – can patients get the care when they need it? If there are delayed discharges, long waiting times, cancelled operations or appointments
Social acceptability	services provided do not meet expectations of patients, service users and the organization. Dignity and privacy are not respected, for example having mixed wards.
Equity	all those in need of the same healthcare do not receive it due to resource allocation or any form of discrimination. In the UK this could relate to the postcode lottery
Relevance	health and social care provided is not relevant to the needs of the community.

(Adapted from Maxwell 1992, Barr and Dowding 2012, Sale 2005)

Table 3.3 Worked example of Maxwell 6: pressure sores

Efficiency and economy	• Time taken to dress wounds increases the workload of staff. • Complications arising due to wound infections, leading to increased time in hospital. • Cost of antibiotics and infection prevention measures required following complications.
Effectiveness	• Lack of assessment, for example using the Norton scale may lead to high-risk groups not being identified early. • Lack of regular turning or protective barriers such as heel protectors. • Failure to refer at-risk patients to the dietician for a review of nutritional levels.
Access	• Failure to apply protective barriers such as heel protectors correctly. • Confused patients removing barriers. This may not be noticed by staff because lower limbs are covered by bed covers.
Social acceptability	• Confused patients not being able to tell staff they are in pain. • Patients with nerve damage not being aware of pressure areas and pain from these. • Increased workloads and prioritization leading to patient voices not being heard. • Lack of candour.
Equity	• Regular turning not being applied. • Protective equipment not being supplied. • Hospital guidelines not being followed.
Relevance	• Hospital processes not being adhered to. • Delays in intervention.

Table 3.3 illustrates an example from practice where the quality of care is affected due to a failure to implement Maxwell's dimensions.

Whilst Maxwell (1992) identifies the importance of these six dimensions, a patient or service user may deem some of the dimensions to be more important than others. For example, the patient or service user may be more concerned with personal aspects such as having their operation cancelled at the last minute, having put childcare in place following surgery they can get to their rehabilitation when needed (*access*). The patient or service user may also be more worried as to whether there will be a long waiting time before their first appointment (*access*). Whereas healthcare professionals may be more focused on whether the general provision is relevant to the needs of the community (*relevance*). Managers will have a more organizational view and therefore may be more concerned with the *efficiency* and *economic* aspects such as, has the best treatment been provided within the resources? Managers may also be more concerned with *effectiveness* – has the evidence base of the intervention been considered?

On the other hand both the patient or service user and healthcare professional may both be concerned with the outcome of an operation (*effectiveness*). However, their reasons may differ. For example, due to rheumatoid arthritis the finger joints may need to be replaced with silicone rubber implants. The patient or service user may in the main be anxious with whether their pain has gone and whether they can carry out their activities of daily living. Whereas the surgeon may be more concerned with the cosmetic outcome of the surgery.

Key point

- Service users, healthcare professionals and managers may have different values.

Dimensions of quality: 3 organizational dimensions

Ovretveit (1992) goes on to argue that there are different perceptions in relation to quality; in other words patients and service users have their own perspective as do healthcare practitioners and managers. If there is conflict between these three, then this impacts on the quality of care. This can be illustrated in figure 3.1.

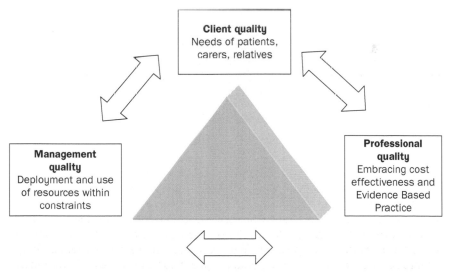

Figure 3.1 Three organizational dimensions. (Adapted from Ovretveit 1992)

Client quality relates to service users being provided with the service that they want. Although individuals generally are better educated today and many have access to the internet, quality care is not like shopping in a supermarket, because clients cannot necessarily choose their healthcare provision. **Professional quality** concerns the viewpoint that the service does meet the needs of the service user as assessed by the professionals. This is because the professionals have the knowledge and skills and understand the evidence base of practice. **Management quality** refers to the resources. Managers hold the budget for all resources and therefore have to use these effectively to meet the service user's needs. One of the complexities of this, though, is that resources are finite.

So, for example, an individual in the UK with multiple sclerosis may read about the effects that cannabis has on spasticity and therefore request this intervention to be provided free of charge on the NHS. However, the professionals may understand that the evidence base linked to this is weak and the managers may consider the cost too high in relation to the number of patients wanting this intervention. This illustrates that there is conflict between these three parties and so care is not considered quality from the patient's perspective.

Key point

- Quality care must not involve conflict between the service user, professional or management.

Another example published in the UK media in 2012, illustrates how some individuals are denied cancer medication due to the high cost of some drugs. This kind of situation also demonstrates conflict between the managers, professionals and patients. The managers and professionals are likely to be focused on the resources involved in cost of treatment and *efficacy* of treatment, whilst the patients want what they see to be the most *effective* treatment. This conflict can result in patients moving home, the media becoming involved and general patient dissatisfaction. In this example, the patient went to the press and treatment was given without his having to move to a different postcode.

Having explored the dimensions of quality that need to be considered, this chapter will now discuss and apply a number of tools that could be used to analyse the causes.

Ishikawa's fishbone

Ishikawa (1985) initiated a simple method that can be used to explain the causes of quality issues through either a root cause analysis or a cause and effect analysis. The aim of this tool is to identify all the causes of the problem systematically, using a fish shape to explore the causes. The problem is illustrated as being in the 'head of the fish' and each cause as being on one of the bones of the fish. This is known as a cause and effect analysis.

If practitioners and patients want to do a more in-depth analysis, the causes of every item listed on the 'bones' are identified separately. For example, figure 3.2 as it stands is a cause and effect diagram. The same diagram can be used as a root cause analysis if all the items listed are discussed, for example the causes of poor lighting, the causes of no British National Formulary (BNF), the causes of interruptions, and so on. So this becomes the root cause analysis in which the analysis is more complex, and so groups may prefer to focus initially on using this tool as a cause and effect tool.

Key points

- The fishbone can be used to analyse causes of quality issues.
- Either a root cause analysis or cause and effect analysis can be completed.

The headings used on the fishbone will depend on the problem being analysed. For example, if you were exploring the reasons behind high staff turnover in a healthcare organization you might choose the following headings:

- economy
- performance of the organization
- organizational culture
- job characteristics
- unrealistic employee expectations and
- personal reasons.

Some often-used headings are

- methods, manpower, materials, machines
- place, policies, people, procedures
- surroundings, suppliers, systems, skills.

To illustrate how the fishbone could be used we have chosen to use the four Ps: place, policies, people and procedures.

Worked examples of Ishikawa's fishbone: medication errors and pressure sores

Chapter 2 discussed the evidence that shows that medication errors and pressure sores are common international quality issues within healthcare practice. The following figures (figure 3.2 and figure 3.3) illustrate two examples from practice related to medication errors and pressure sores and show how the fishbone could be used to explain the reasons why these quality issues may occur within practice.

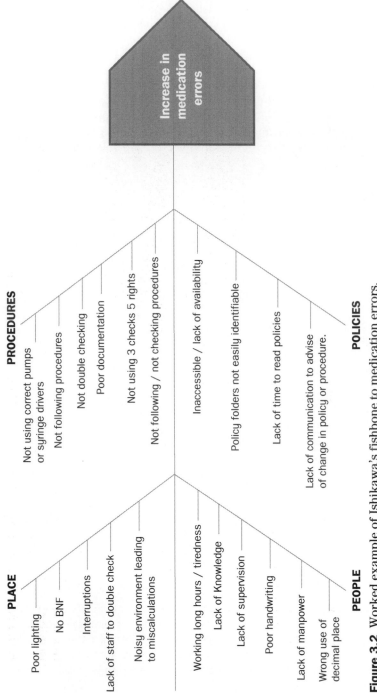

Figure 3.2 Worked example of Ishikawa's fishbone to medication errors.

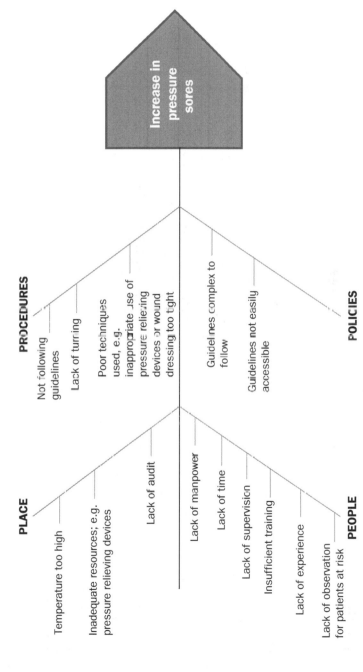

Figure 3.3 Worked example of Ishikawa's fishbone to pressure sores.

Activity

Reflect on a quality issue from your practice:

- Draw a fishbone and analyse the reasons that could be used to explain why this issue arises.
- Begin with a cause and effect fishbone and then take some of the 'causes' and think about the 'root' causes.

There are a number of strengths and limitations of the fishbone and these are illustrated in table 3.4.

Table 3.4 Strengths and limitations of Ishikawa's fishbone

Strengths	Limitations
- Visual presentation. - Can be used as both a cause and effect and root cause analysis. - Simple tool to use. - Identifies causes of quality issues.	- Due to simplicity of the cause–effect analysis wider issues could get missed. - Does not provide the solutions. - Does not prioritize which problems need to be resolved first.

SWOT

Another tool that could be used within the quality circle is SWOT (strengths, weaknesses, opportunities and threats). This is a well-known tool developed by Ansoff (1987, cited in Barr and Dowding 2012) which has been around for over 40 years, that could be used to explore the causes of quality issues. Using this tool can be an inclusive process in that staff and other stakeholders (service users, carers) can be involved in the analysis.

Chambers et al. (2004) highlight that the weaknesses could also be viewed as challenges, and Walshe and Smith (2011) acknowledge that some individuals may perceive strengths as weaknesses and opportunities as threats, and vice versa. Two key aspects that are generally applied when using this tool are that the S and W relate to the *internal* factors that impact on organizational outcomes and the O and T relate to the *external* factors that could be outside practitioners' control but nevertheless impact on the organization (Sale 2005, Swage 2004). However, Barr and Dowding (2012) do not make this distinction between the internal and external factors. Unlike Ishikawa's fishbone, a SWOT analysis will explore the wider aspects, that is, the strengths as well as the weaknesses and the opportunities as well as the threats.

Key points

- SWOT can be used to identify the internal and external factors impacting on quality care.
- SWOT demonstrates that not all factors are within an individual's control.

Once the factors have been listed, then each point can be discussed in relation to possible clinical governance strategies that can be used to resolve the various factors.

Activity

Thinking about a specific quality issue in your workplace:

- What are the strengths and weaknesses?
- What might be the opportunities and threats?

When undertaking a SWOT analysis and thinking about the strengths and weaknesses, Chambers et al. (2004:94) highlight a number of points for practitioners to consider, and you may have thought about the following questions in the previous activity:

- Do staff currently employed in the organization have up-to-date knowledge and skills in relation to their area of practice?
- If not, is continuing professional development accessible for all staff? Are opportunities for further learning provided and resourced?
- Do professionals understand and value the different roles within the organization?
- Is communication within the organization effective?
- Do staff have good time management, organizational skills and problem-solving, decision-making skills?

When thinking about the opportunities and threats outside the practitioner's control, the following questions may be helpful:

- What potential career pathways could be implemented?
- What interests could be developed?
- Are there any barriers to implementing continuing professional development?
- What impact does local or national policy have on change?

In order for a SWOT analysis to be effective it is essential for organizations and teams to identify an action plan that should detail how the strengths could be developed further, how the weaknesses could be surmounted, how the organization could make the most of the opportunities and how the threats could be limited (Walshe and Smith 2011) or turned into opportunities.

Worked examples using SWOT: falls in the older population and Ventilator-Acquired Pneumonia

As discussed in chapter 2, falls in the older population is an internationally common occurrence and impacts on the quality of care provided. Tables 3.5 and 3.6 identify examples from practice.

Table 3.5 Application of SWOT – falls

Strengths	Weaknesses
• Equipment: up-to-date hoists, chairs, footwear, bedrails, low/high beds. • Experienced staff (length of service in area at least three years): 50% of staff. • Incident reporting: staff are good at reporting falls, which helps to reduce falls. • Policies readily available.	• Poor falls assessment of patient on admission by nurses (looks at patient's past medical history, balance, mental capacity, medication, if there is postural drop and incontinence). • Is the falls assessment tool used adequate? Oliver and Healey (2009) state that most tools aren't tested for validity and reliability. • Ward too busy for adequate patient falls assessment. • Lack of understanding of importance of assessment from staff due to lack of knowledge. • No care plan put in place when patient is identified as at risk of falls. • Shortage of staff: less staff per patient. • Environment: slippery floors at times, poor lighting, cluttered area around bed space, patient isn't always nursed in most appropriate place on ward (too far away from nurse station) • Equipment: available, but not always used. • Inexperienced staff (newly qualified, little experience in the area): 50%
Opportunities	**Threats**
• Professional development: university modules courses, e-learning courses (mandatory: slips and falls). • New technology: movement alarms and hip protectors available. • Education and training: to highlight weaknesses.	• Staff shortages due to government cuts (recently less overlap between shifts). • Limited money for staff training. • Aging population increasing. • Complex, multiple diagnoses. • Policies: evidence may not be up to date. • Limited resources.

Table 3.6 Application of SWOT – Ventilator Associated Pneumonia (VAP is a nosocomial airway infection and is associated with increased ITU [Intensive Therapy Unit] and hospital stays and also has significantly increased costs [Safdar et al. 2005])

Strengths	Weaknesses
• VAP Care Bundles as a means to deliver Evidence Based Practice and to measure compliance. • Teaching on VAPs on mandatory study days for nursing staff. • Having the right equipment on the unit, e.g. mouth foam swabs for Chlorhexidine application, electric beds to sit the patient up 30–45 degrees. • Supportive ward manager. • Member of staff belonging to the Thames Valley Critical Care Network (an action group who discuss auditing of care bundles and preventative measures).	• Nursing cultures – deficiencies in clinical practice and working in certain ways that misses key points identified to reduce VAPs. • Staff resistant to change to new recommended practice. • Staff/patients disliking impregnated toothbrushes used in our unit. • Monthly care bundle audit results demonstrating low compliance on mouth-care practice as a preventative measure for VAP. • Lack of knowledge and/or education on VAPs for some staff. • The VAP care bundle needs to be used in combination of all the elements all of the time to have greater effect on the positive outcome; audits reveal that it is not. • Lack of medical lead/interest to help drive the prevention of VAPs.
Opportunities	**Threats**
• Department of Health's Saving Lives Programme including high impact interventions to reduce hospital acquired infections such as VAPs. • Thames Valley Critical Care Network – Quarterly meetings; representative from each unit to attend their meetings. • New technologies with ventilation, different ventilation modes to improve lung compliance. Availability of Extracorporeal Membrane Oxygenation from other units for severe pneumonias. • NICE patient safety guidelines for ventilated patients.	• Cost implications/limitations of resources needed to help reduce VAPs, e.g. endotracheal tubes with subglottic aspiration ports, continuous cuff measurement manometers. • Ageing population and increased ITU admissions with co-morbidities – more likely to develop VAP.

Activity

Reflect on your practice.

- Use the same quality issue that you chose to apply to Ishikawa's fishbone.
- Draw a table and identify the factors in each quadrant that could be used to explain the causes of this issue.
- Does this tool provide you with more information to consider than Ishikawa's fishbone?
- What would you consider the strengths and limitations of SWOT to be?

SWOT is also a useful tool for individuals to use in relation to their own personal development.

Activity

Thinking about your role at work, use SWOT to identify your personal strengths, weaknesses or challenges, opportunities and threats. We suggest you draw a table with four quadrants, as illustrated above.
   The following questions may guide you:

- Begin with the positives! What are you good at?
- What knowledge and skills would you like to develop within the next five years?
- Are there any barriers that would prevent you achieving your goals?
- What opportunities are there within your organization or external to your organization?

Once this table is completed, you may like to discuss your findings with your line manager. Having completed the table and having discussed it with your manager, it is not the end of the process because no doubt an action plan will need to be formulated, and this will include change. Change can be challenging and the management of change will be discussed and applied in the following chapter.

Key points

- Individuals can use SWOT for personal development.
- Teams can analyse causes of quality issues using SWOT.

Although SWOT is a useful tool, there are a number of limitations as well as strengths to consider, some of which are identified in table 3.7.

Table 3.7 Critique of SWOT

Strengths	Limitations
• Guides thinking. • Considers the wider picture. • Results can facilitate strategic planning. • Can be linked to audit and the results can increase motivation. • Can be used individually for career development or within teams to analyse problems. • Weaknesses can be addressed to improve the efficiency and economy of the organization – this links back to Maxwell 6. • Weaknesses can be developed into strengths. • Threats can be turned into Opportunities. • Can be used for individual development, team and organizational development.	• Strategic decisions are not evident from the list provided. • Highlighting weaknesses could be considered challenging to staff. • Could be considered too simplistic. • Does not provide the resolutions. • Does not help teams to prioritize. • Organizations cannot necessarily influence the threats, e.g. government legislation.

(Adapted from Barr and Dowding 2012, Chambers et al. 2004, Sale 2005, Swage 2004 and Swayne et al. 2010)

PESTLE/PEST

This tool explores how the Political, Economic, Social, Technical, Legal and Environmental factors could be used to understand factors leading to poor quality care. Teams may prefer to use PEST and this could be due to a preference of not exploring the legal and ethical factors. The example given later in this chapter illustrates PEST. PESTLE may be used to further analyse the issues highlighted by SWOT (Swage 2004). For example, when analysing the opportunities or threats of the organization, the PESTLE acronym could be used to guide thinking regarding what political, economic and social factors, and so on, could be deemed to threaten the organization. However, this tool explores only the external factors impacting on the quality of care, unlike SWOT, which considers both the internal and external factors.

Teams could consider what local and national *political* government initiatives hinder healthcare organizational objectives or how local patient lobby groups affect service provision. Looking at the *economic* factors, healthcare provision could be affected through financial constraints at either local or national levels. In chapter 1 we discussed the impact of *social* factors in relation to the impact that changing demographics have on service provision and the quality of care. *Technological* changes occur at a fast pace and so if staff are not provided with the required training, this can impact on the quality of care provided. PESTLE can be used to help organizations analyse the current situation as well as helping to plan for future developments.

In chapter 2 we discussed needle stick injuries. NSIs are associated with a small but significant risk to a healthcare professional's career, health, family and, of course, patients (Pathak et al. 2011). Between 1997 and 2008 a total of 3773 blood-born virus exposure incidents involving healthcare workers were reported to the Health Protection Agency (HPA 2008). Table 3.8 illustrates how PEST could be used to examine the external factors.

Table 3.8 Worked example of PEST – needle stick injuries

Political	• New legislation not followed, such as Health and Safety – Sharps Instruments in Healthcare – Regulations 2013 (Implemented in the EU Council Directive 2010/32/EU). • Failure to meet external standards set by NICE. • Poor workforce planning leading to insufficient skill mix.
Economic	• Pressure of healthcare costs leading to a lack of sharps bins. • Rising cost of resources leading to a lack of manpower and therefore increased risk of needle stick injuries occurring.
Social	• Higher expectations from the public. • Lack of role models leading to staff taking short cuts and risks, for example re-sheathing (recapping) needles. • Change in demographics leading to increased use of healthcare services.
Technological	• New devices available but not necessarily purchased.

As with all tools there are strengths and limitations of using this one. Table 3.9 illustrates some of these.

Table 3.9 Critique of PEST(LE)

Strengths	Limitations
• Encourages strategic thinking. • Provides a wider understanding of issues. • Raises awareness of possible threats to an organization. • Provides greater depth than a SWOT analysis.	• External factors are dynamic and change quickly. • Does not encourage critical examination of the factors. • A useful PEST requires a lot of information to be collected and this is not possible in a table. • The data need to be accurate and timely.

> **Activity**
>
> - Compare and contrast Ishikawa's fishbone, SWOT and PEST/PESTLE.
> - Can you think of any further advantages or disadvantages?
> - Do you have a preference for one of the tools and, if so, why?

Key point summary

There are a number of ways that quality issues may be analysed. These include Maxwell 6, the 3 Organizational Dimensions, Ishikawa's fishbone, SWOT and PESTLE, and there are strengths and limitations to all of these tools. There is no prescribed tool for a particular quality issue and so a team could decide to use Ishikawa's fishbone because they like to see a visual representation of the issue. Whereas another team may choose SWOT, to encourage them to consider both external and internal factors.

- Quality circles enable healthcare teams and service users to work together to analyse quality issues. Managers, service users and healthcare professionals meet to share ideas, prioritize areas for improvement and agree solutions using clinical governance strategies.
- According to Maxwell (1984, 1992) quality consists of six dimensions: efficiency and economy, effectiveness, access, social acceptability, equity, relevance. If there are issues with any of these dimensions, Maxwell considers that a quality issue has arisen.
- Ovretveit (1992) argues that client quality, professional quality and management quality need to be in alignment.
- Ishikawa's fishbone is used to identify the causes of a problem systematically. This can be used in its simplest form as a cause and effect analysis or a more detailed root cause analysis.
- SWOT encourages examination of internal and external factors impacting on quality care.
- PESTLE/PEST is useful when examining the macroenvironment.

Implications for practice

- Practitioners and service users need to work together to ensure that the quality of health and social care continues to improve.
- Practitioners need to understand the different dimensions that could impact on quality care.
- Practitioners need to select an appropriate tool to analyse quality issues, based on the summary above.

- Whichever analysis is used, it is key that teams agree an action plan. Teams also need to identify possible clinical governance strategies that could be used to improve the quality of healthcare provision.

End-of-chapter questions

- How do quality circles differ from focus groups?
- Which would appear to be your preferred tool?

See the Appendix on page 192 for suggested answers to these questions.

References

Ansoff H (1987) *Corporate strategy.* London: Penguin

Barr J and Dowding L (2012) *Leadership in health care.* London: Sage

Chambers R, Tavabie A, Mohanna K, Wakley G (2004) *The good appraisal toolkit for primary care.* Oxford: Radcliffe

Directive 2010/32/EU Prevention from sharp injuries in the hospital and healthcare sector. Available at https://www.osha.europa.eu/en/legislation/directives/sector-specific-and-worker-related-provisions/osh-dirctives/council-directive-2010-32-eu (accessed 30.03.2013)

Health Protection Agency Centre for Infections, National Public Health Service for Wales, CDSC Northern Ireland and Health Protection Scotland (2008) *Eye of the Needle: Surveillance of significant occupational exposure to blood borne viruses in healthcare workers.* London: HPA

Ishikawa K (1985) *What is total quality control? The Japanese Way.* Harlow: Prentice Hall

Keleman M (2005) *Managing quality.* London: Sage

Maxwell R (1984) Quality assessment in health. *British Medical Journal,* May 288, 1470–1472

Maxwell R (1992) Dimensions of quality revisited: From thought to action. *Quality in Healthcare,* 1, 171–177

Moullin M (2002) *Delivering excellence in health and social care.* Maidenhead: Open University Press

Mullins L (2010) *Management and organisational behaviour.* London: Prentice Hall

Oliver D and Healey F (2009) Falls risk prediction tools for hospital inpatients: Do they work? *Nursing Times,* 105 (7), 18–21

Ovretveit (1992) *Health service quality.* Oxford: Blackwell Scientific

Pathak R, Kahlon KH, Ahluwalia SK, Sharma S, Bhardwaj R (2011) Needle stick injury and inadequate post exposure practices among healthcare workers in a tertiary care centre in rural India. *International Journal of Collaborative Research on Internal Medicine and Public Health,* 4 (5), 638

Safdar N, Saint S, Collard H, Dezfulian C (2005) Clinical and economic consequences of ventilator-associated pneumonia: A systematic review. *Critical Care Medicine,* 33, 1582–1583

Sale D (2005) *Understanding clinical governance and quality assurance: Making it happen*. Basingstoke: Palgrave Macmillan

Swage T (2004) *Clinical governance in healthcare practice*. London: Butterworth Heinemann

Swayne L, Duncan W and Ginter P (2010) *Strategic management of healthcare organisations*. Chichester: Jossey-Bass

Walshe K and Smith J (2011) *Healthcare management*. Maidenhead: Open University Press

4

Developing clinical governance strategies through change management

Mary Gottwald and Gail E Lansdown

Chapter contents

- Learning objectives
- Introduction
- Barriers to change
- Managing resistance
- Transition period for change
- Developmental, transitional and transformational change
- Diffusion of innovations model of change
- The RAID model of change
- Lewin's Force-Field Analysis model of change
- The four A's model of change
- Key point summary
- Implications for practice
- End-of-chapter questions
- References

Learning objectives

By the end of this chapter, the reader will be better able to

- understand the barriers to change
- apply four models of change to workplace issues.

'Change is not made without inconvenience, even from worse to better' (Richard Hooker [1554–1600], British theologian. Quoted in Samuel Johnson, *Dictionary of the English Language*, preface [1755]).

Introduction

This chapter will highlight some of the challenges and obstacles impacting on change and discuss how change agents, advocacy groups, involvement of patients and service users can ensure the smooth transition of change. There are a plethora of change management models, and this chapter will consider the Diffusion of Innovation, the RAID model, four A's of change and Lewin's Force-Field Analysis.

In order for health and social care practitioners to continually develop and improve the quality of care provided, there is bound to be a need for change. Management of change, therefore, is an essential skill for healthcare professionals to have and this can also help to ensure that the implementation of clinical governance strategies occurs. Healthcare changes rapidly and is continuously changing (Carnall 2007) with 85% of healthcare organizations undergoing transformational change every two years. Successful operation in this arena requires the successful management of change and good leadership.

Healthcare changes rapidly and is continuously changing, and therefore it is essential that healthcare professionals develop their abilities to constantly adapt to organizational change (Beerel 2009). Parkin (2009:9) describes change as a 'phenomenon of daily organisational life', so one thing that we can be sure about is that in order to improve the quality of health and social care provision we will frequently need to be involved in change initiatives. Changing practice to improve patient care can only be seen as a positive outcome. However, there are barriers to change initiatives, and therefore, in order to avoid conflict, managers and leaders of change need to manage both the change, that is, the situation, and the staff who are affected by the change (Sullivan and Garland 2013).

Barriers to change

Response to change initiatives varies and ranges from complete engagement and acceptance of the change to total resistance. In this chapter we will be discussing the more commonly presented barriers to change such as resistance to change, disempowerment, uncertainty and loss. However, first of all it is necessary to think about the factors that influence nurses to raise concerns about quality of care and standards of practice through whistle-blowing.

Whistle-blowing

As stated by Attree (2007), although under-reported, nurses are required by their professional body to raise concerns about quality of care. However, the fear of repercussions, reprisals, labelling (as whistle-blowers) and blame for raising concerns prevent them from reporting. Reporting is seen as a high risk/low benefit action, and Attree (2007) concludes that, in order to promote a culture of openness, which in turn promotes quality and learning, the barriers to reporting concerns need to be removed.

This is further supported by Jackson et al. (2010), who in their article investigate via semi-structured interviews the reasons why nurses blow the whistle and their consequent experience of being whistle-blowers. They identified that the participants in their study found the experience to be highly stressful, with three main themes occurring:

1. Reasons for whistle-blowing: 'I just couldn't advocate.'
2. Feeling silenced: 'Nobody speaks out.'
3. Climate of fear: 'You are just not safe.'

Although the nurses felt they were acting as required by their professional body, as stated earlier by Attree (2007), they felt there was a need for clarity about how they were expected to act as the patients' advocate, that clear guidelines about how to raise concerns were needed, that systems needed to react quickly and appropriately to concerns raised by nurses and that an environment of safety in which to raise concerns needed to be promoted.

Activity

- Has it been necessary for you to be a whistle-blower?
- How did your colleagues respond to this action?
- How did your organization respond to this action?

Resistance to change

For some individuals, changing practice is not a challenge. They see change as an invigorating and positive experience and therefore these individuals will drive the change forward (Sullivan and Garland 2013). However, change can be a complex process and there is evidence to suggest that some healthcare professionals find managing change challenging due to employee resistance to change initiatives (McSherry and Pearce 2002, Sullivan and Garland 2013).

Parkin (2009:155) asserts that resistance is 'where change implementers perceive a difficulty in having their ideas as accepted or the change is thwarted or sabotaged by others'. This resistance could become a barrier to the successful implementation of clinical governance strategies. Carnall (2007:3) questions whether 'this resistance to change is really resistance to uncertainty'. The resistance is not due to the 'change' per se but due to the individual's uncertainty about the process. For example, individuals could be concerned that they may lose their status and incur a loss of salary and therefore may become hesitant to engage in change behaviour.

Key point

- Resistance to change is a normal part of any change initiative

Activity

- Reflect for a moment upon a change that took place within your own organization.
- Reflect on your own reaction to this change.
- How did this make you feel in the beginning?
- How did you react?
- Did your feelings change over a period of time?

Activity

- Consider why some staff in your team resist and challenge change initiatives.
- Make a list of the barriers to change.

You may have considered some of the following barriers to change:

1. Staff may feel the change could reduce their level of power or influence and so they may feel personal loss, for example loss of self-esteem. They may also feel undermined.
2. Staff may go through a period of uncertainty, for example they may feel that they will not be able to meet the new demands of their jobs. This is all linked to loss of control, loss of predictability and fear of the unknown.
3. Expectations may differ, and the benefits of change could be seen to be biased towards one group's needs at the expense of another group. For example, if the change is seen to benefit the management structure within the organization whilst increasing the workload for the workforce, then there is likely to be resistance to the change process.
4. Anything that requires the individual to readjust to their environment can cause stress and resistance. Individuals may use 'denial' as a defence mechanism; however, this should be considered a normal, healthy reaction to organizational change.
5. Staff may not have been included in discussions linked to change. They may therefore feel that important information has not been communicated and managers are not empathetic towards their concerns as well as their individual issues. There may be misunderstanding and distrust, for example if the working relationship between manager and staff is tense and the manager initiates the change (top-down approach), then staff may resist due to lack of trust. It is essential that the leader/manager ensures the team are up to date with what is going on.

Chambers et al. (2007), Kotter and Schlesinger (2008) and Sullivan and Garland (2013) identify further barriers such as a lack of trust, a lack of understanding of the need for a particular change and therefore a lack of consensus, a lack of resources and a lack of evidence for the need for change or simply because they dislike the person initiating and managing the change. Kotter and Schlesinger (2008) also suggest that leaders and managers simply do not take the time to explore and understand the reasons why staff resist the change.

Key points

- Leaders of change must consider the barriers.
- Staff need to be supported through the change process.

Managing resistance

Kotter and Schlesinger (2008:5) suggest the four key methods below could be used to manage resistance.

Education and communication

One of the barriers considered earlier was lack of communication and involvement in discussions surrounding change initiatives. Change agents could help staff understand the rationale for change through team discussions; one-to-one discussions, staff development workshops or presentations. Having a clear action plan also ensures that staff understand the time frames and pace of change.

Participation and involvement

Change agents could take a more participative approach and involve teams in devising the change initiative and drawing up the action plan suggested above. By involving teams in the decision-making process there is more likely to be a feeling of ownership. However, this participative approach could be seen to be more time consuming and not realistic if the change initiative needs to be implemented quickly.

Facilitation and support

Providing education and training has already been mentioned above. Adapting to change involves emotional responses, and so a key attribute for the change agents is to have good 'listening' skills. The Human Resource department may need to provide counsellors to talk with staff who are feeling overwhelmed or having difficulties adjusting to change.

Negotiation and agreement

This is a particularly important aspect when the change initiative impacts on an individual's role, because any impact on role identity will result in defensiveness and this would be a barrier to a change initiative. Therefore this links back to the previous discussion on the importance of communication.

Transition period for change

Change takes time and therefore the leaders and managers of change (change agents) not only have to recognize potential resistance but must remember that teams will be going through a transition period. A number of changes to self-esteem can take place during this period. Hence it is imperative to acknowledge this and to support colleagues during a change initiative, as at any one time each member could be in a different stage of the transition period (figure 4.1). It is particularly important for those in a management and leadership role to remember this. Barr and Dowding (2012) liken change to Kubler Ross's (1969) five stage grieving process (denial, anger, bargaining, depression and acceptance).

Activity

- Click on the following link to read more about the five stages of the grieving process http://www.businessballs.com/elisabeth_kubler_ross_five_stages_of_grief.htm
- Look back at the notes you made when reflecting upon a change that took place within your own organization.
- Were some of your feelings similar to these five stages?

Changes In self-esteem during periods of transition

Figure 4.1 illustrates seven stages that individuals may go through when faced with the challenges of change. There is no time frame associated with each stage, and so when working with your colleagues it is important to consider that some staff may take longer to move through the stages and therefore could do with some support, whilst others progress more quickly. Whilst, for some, change can be an exciting and motivating experience, for others change causes anxiety.

Key points

- Staff need to be aware that others may be struggling during periods of transition.
- Staff need to support each other during periods of transition.

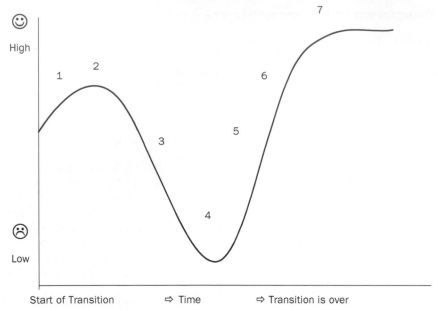

1. *Numbness*: Staff may not understand the reason behind the change and may feel 'shocked' and unable to reason and make plans. Those who feel positive about the need for change will find this stage less intense.
2. *Denial/minimization*: Changes needed may be minimized and staff may feel that the changes required are not as bad as expected. However, this could be due to defence mechanisms being used.
3. *Self-doubt*: The realities of change are now more evident, and as staff become more aware they may feel uncertainty and self-doubt. However, this stage also has high-energy periods for some.
4. *Acceptance of reality/letting go*: Moving through the first three stages has still involved some attachment to the past. This fourth stage involves 'letting go' and is often a stage of optimism.
5. *Testing*: Staff become much more active, trying out new behaviours and ways of coping with the transition and change.
6. *Search for meaning*: There is much more understanding of the changes needed within the organization. Once staff have understood how the changes affect their roles within the organization, they are able to move to the final stage.
7. *Internalization*: The changes are accepted and become part of the daily routine and practice. At this point staff become more positive, and begin to build on the new strengths they have developed.

Figure 4.1 Stages of transition. (Adapted from: Hopson et al. 2000)

Developmental, transitional and transformational change

Barr and Dowding (2012) and Iles and Sutherland (2001) identify three kinds of change:

1. Developmental change
2. Transitional change
3. Transformational change.

Developmental change

Developmental change can be seen to improve the effectiveness of current practice within the organization, for example the focus of change could be the implementation of care bundles (discussed further in chapter 7) and the skills and processes required to implement care bundles. It may be *planned* (deliberate) or *emergent* (sometimes unfolds in a natural, spontaneous and unplanned way) (Iles and Sutherland 2001).

Planned change may occur as a result of external political, economic, social or technical factors impacting on the organization (Mullins 2010). These external factors would be clearly demonstrated through the use of a PEST analysis. This change may occur because of an intended change by the change agent, and therefore leaders, as the change agents in healthcare, need to think about and plan the changes carefully. They must ensure that the change occurs at the right time, is relevant and impacts positively on staff, patients and service users. If leaders communicate and involve staff, patients and service users in this planned change, then there is likely to be less resistance (Iles and Sutherland 2001, Barr and Dowding 2012).

Emergent change could be seen as a more 'bottom-up' approach where frontline staff constantly problem-solve together, implementing a range of solutions (Parkin 2009), and therefore the change takes place automatically.

Transitional change

Transitional change (figure 4.2) involves the implementation of something different. It can be episodic, planned or a radical organizational change, such

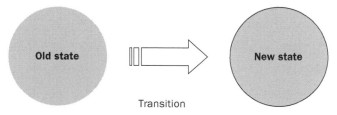

Transition

Figure 4.2 Transitional change. (Iles and Sutherland 2001:16)

as, for example, in April 2013 the move in the UK from Primary Care Trusts to Clinical Commissioning Groups who are now the commissioners of most National Health Services in England. Management of the interim transition state is needed over a controlled period of time (Iles and Sunderland 2001, Barr and Dowding 2012), as staff will be going through the stages of transition as outlined in figure 4.1.

Transformational change

Transformational change (figure 4.3) is an emergence of a new state, unknown until it takes shape. The time taken for this change is not easily controlled and it is a major organizational change of structures, processes and the culture within organizations (Iles and Sunderland 2001, Barr and Dowding 2008).

For example, the accident and emergency team may identify that having an acute admissions unit would improve the patient's experience. The initiation of an acute admissions unit linked to the accident and emergency department but functioning as a separate department could help reduce the four hour waiting time. The new acute admissions unit would act as a gateway between the GP, the emergency department and the wards of the hospital and therefore improve collaboration. However, for this to happen, consideration would need to be given to the structures, processes and culture within the organization.

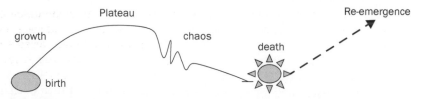

Figure 4.3 Transformational change. (Iles and Sutherland 2001:16)

Whatever the nature of the change, Kotter and Schlesinger (2008) suggest that there are three key steps to implementing successful change, and models of change used must facilitate this:

1. Analysing the situational factors.
2. Agreeing the most favourable pace of change.
3. Considering how resistance to change will be managed.

Key points

- Change may be planned or emergent.
- Change may be episodic or radical.
- It can take time to adapt to new changes.

Models of change

There are a number of models that could be used within change management to support teams applying the principles of clinical governance. Four will be discussed here in this second section of the chapter:

1. Diffusion of innovation theory.
2. RAID.
3. Lewin's Force-Field Analysis.
4. The four A's of change.

Regardless of the change model chosen, there are three basic aspects to consider for all models:

1. Recognition of the need to change.
2. Implementation of an action plan for change (goals and strategies).
3. A period of consolidation and evaluation.

Diffusion of innovations model of change

Diffusion is defined as 'The process by which an innovation is communicated through certain channels over time among members of a social system. It is a special type of communication, in that the messages are concerned with new ideas' (Rogers 1983:5).

At a simplistic level, this is about the ways that are used to communicate new ideas and changes to practice. If the idea is perceived by change agents (policymakers, leaders and managers) as being *new*, then it is considered an *innovation*. When innovative ideas are adopted and diffused, resulting in outcomes, then social change has transpired (Rogers 1983). This model works in two ways in that healthcare teams may adopt the change but then decide to revert to the original practice or may initially reject the proposed change but then adopt it at a later date. Rogers (1983 cited in Sullivan and Garland 2013:195) identifies five steps to this model:

1. *Knowledge*: The proposed change is communicated to staff so that they have an understanding of the change and rationale behind the change.
2. *Persuasion*: Staff may be either for or against the proposed change.
3. *Decision*: Teams collaborate and discuss the change in order either to adopt or not adopt it.
4. *Implementation*: The new change is implemented and the strengths and limitations of the innovation evaluated. Further changes may occur following evaluation.
5. *Confirmation*: If the innovation is considered positive and successful following evaluation, then change continues; otherwise the innovation is rejected. If unsuccessful, the innovator may then decide to review the initiative and implement it at a later date.

Sullivan and Garland (2013) identify one disadvantage of this model in that it is imperative for the innovators to have the support of policymakers, leaders and managers within the organization because without this the proposed change is not likely to succeed.

According to Rogers (1983:21) in the main, these five steps must occur in a '...time-ordered sequence of knowledge, persuasion, decision, implementation, and confirmation. The *innovation–decision period* is the length of time required to pass through the innovation–decision period process.'

Table 4.1 identifies some strengths and limitations of the Diffusion of Innovation model.

Table 4.1 Critique of Diffusion of Innovation model

Strengths	Limitations
• Focuses on new ideas and innovative practice • Allows flexibility in adoption or rejection of proposed innovative change • Allows teams to progress through stages before final adoption of the innovation • Recognizes that equal numbers of individuals are either for or against adopting the change • If change is rejected, the model allows innovator to make alterations to proposed change and revive the innovation	• Requires commitment and support of policymakers, leaders and managers • Getting a new idea adopted is difficult due to uncertainty • Adopting innovations can be a lengthy process • Requires effective and clear two-way communication

(Rogers 1983, Sullivan and Garland 2013)

We have already discussed how some individuals are enthusiastic and adopt the change quickly and in a positive manner, whereas others are more resistant to change and take longer to adopt new process, structures and procedures. Table 4.2 illustrates how Rogers (1983) uses a specific system for classifying adopters, based on the time it takes to adopt new innovative ideas.

Activity

Refer back to the first activity in this chapter where you reflected on a change that occurred in your organization.

Questions for you to consider:

• Would you consider this change to be innovative? Reflect on the rationale for your answer.

- In your organization and/or team, who would you consider to be the *innovators, early adopters or early majority?*
- Was this change successfully implemented due to the *innovators, early adopters or early majority?*
- What did these early adopters do to make the change process smooth and successful?
- In your organization and/or team, who would you consider to be the *late majority and laggards.*
- Did the *late majority and laggards* impact on the implementation of this change?
- Why did these late adopters resist the change?

The RAID model of change

The RAID model (Figure 4.4: Review, Agreement, Implementation and Demonstration) has been used within UK NHS organizations successfully and was developed by the National Clinical Governance Support Team (Bull and Veall 2009). According to Rogers (2006:79), 'the experiences of patients and staff have been improved by the teams who have used the RAID approach to bring about change'.

According to Rogers (2006) and Bull and Veall (2009) the strengths of this cyclical model are that

1. It allows creativity and innovation and facilitates a 'bottom-up' approach

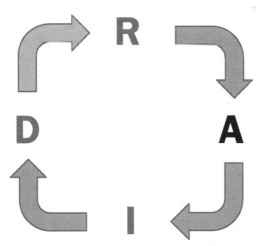

Figure 4.4 The RAID model. (Adapted from Rogers 2006:74)

2. It fosters continuous education and training of staff to enable and motivate them to maintain continuous changes to their practice.

RAID is based on the acceptance that those who are delivering and managing healthcare services, as well as those receiving healthcare services, are involved in the decision-making. This therefore differs from a 'top-down' hierarchical approach. This does not mean to say that managers should not be included; in fact their support is vital. If managers, ward managers, front line staff, patients and service users communicate and collaborate, then this is more likely to lead to a change initiative such as the implementation of clinical governance strategies being effective. However, involvement in decision-making is not sufficient and Bull and Veall (2009) emphasize that another advantage of this model is that it fosters constant education and training of staff to enable and motivate them to maintain continuous changes to their practice. Figure 1.4 (chapter 1) illustrates how education and training are one of the key clinical governance strategies.

In order to review the challenges, achievements and implement any change process, good communication skills and listening skills are vital (Bishop 2010) during all stages of this model.

Stage 1: Review

The first stage of this model involves a working group to review the current service both at a local and national level. This review involves the gathering of information from those in management positions, clinical and non-clinical staff, service users, carers and families (Rogers 2006), and therefore supports the Haxby et al. (2010) definition of service user involvement that we discussed in chapter 1. One of the advantages of including a varied group is that those who are directly affected by the change can be involved from the beginning. They can share their experiences of the current service provision and can also have a say in any planned changes, thus having a 'sense of ownership' (Rogers 2006:75). This supports the notion that RAID is a 'bottom-up' model of change. The final part of this stage is for the team to suggest potential recommendations demonstrating how changes and improvements to the quality of service provision will be achieved.

Stage 2: Agree

During this stage of this model, the review panel agrees on specific actions and changes. Those at the top of the organization and those involved in the review need to be confident that the proposed changes support the organization's strategic direction. Managers have to ensure that any changes to the service do not negatively impact on other services. At the more local level, teams will have to ensure that changes are prioritized and operationalized. It is not necessarily possible to implement all recommendations in one go and therefore teams will have to prioritize and perhaps select changes that are easy to implement successfully without too many resources (Rogers 2006).

Stage 3: Implement

This stage involves recommendations being actioned and requires strong leadership. Leaders need to identify the agenda, timetable and actions required in order to implement the recommendations (Rogers 2006). Barr and Dowding (2012) suggest that the GANNT chart (developed by Gannt in the early twentieth century), commonly used within healthcare practice and easily downloaded from the internet is used to draw up this timetable.

Stage 4: Demonstrate

As with all models of change, this stage involves evaluation. If some aspects of the change process are deemed to have been unsuccessful, then teams can discuss lessons learned and reflect on actions to be taken to develop current strategies. It is essential that the results of the evaluation are disseminated to the members of the original review group as well as the employees of the organization. Patients and service users may wish to communicate successful changes using the Patient Voices Programme mentioned in chapter 1.

Worked example from practice: diabetes care (Bull and Veall 2009)

Figure 4.5 illustrates how the RAID model was used in practice to increase the number of link-nurses working with individuals with diabetes as well as working with secondary care nurses, their families and carers. We can see that the key clinical governance strategy implemented in this worked example is *education and training* and this strategy will be discussed in more depth in the next chapter.

Aims of project

- To increase the number and motivation of secondary care link-nurses within the district general hospital site.
- To enhance their knowledge and bridge the theory–practice gap in dissemination of that knowledge (Bull and Veall 2009:300).

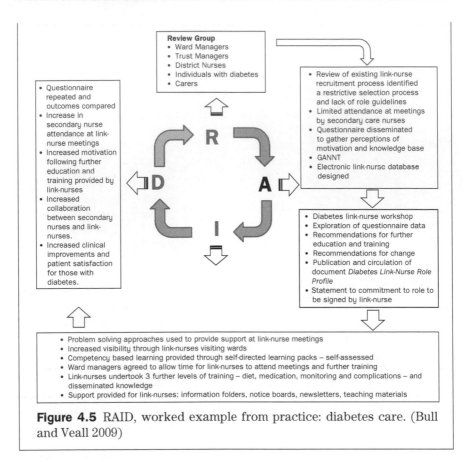

Figure 4.5 RAID, worked example from practice: diabetes care. (Bull and Veall 2009)

In this worked example, the application of the RAID model was successful because

1. A bottom-up approach was used
2. Support for link-nurses was provided through education and training
3. This increased their knowledge in relation to diabetes care
4. The impact of this was that these link-nurses were then able to disseminate their knowledge to nurses involved in the care of those with diabetes
5. This in turn led to improved care and service user/patient satisfaction.

Key points

- RAID involves managers, front-line staff, patients and carers.
- RAID is a bottom-up approach.
- RAID facilitates change and improves service delivery and quality care.

Activity

- Consider your own area of practice.
- Reflect on your target population and choose one group, for example stroke, substance misuse.
- Consider an issue where the quality of care could be improved for this group.
- Refer back to figure 4.4 and, taking each stage in turn (*review, agreement, implementation and demonstration*), consider how this model could be used to manage the change process and resolve your quality issue.
- Who would you involve in the review group?
- How could you go about applying this model to practice?

All models have their strengths and limitation and some of these are highlighted in table 4.2

Table 4.2 Critique of the RAID model

Strengths	Limitations
• A 'bottom-up' model • Engages service users and staff in quality improvement programmes • Identifies key projects for teams to engage with • Allows creativity and innovation (Rogers 2006) • Encourages problem-solving • Motivates staff to continually develop the quality of healthcare provision • Fosters continuous professional development through education and training.	• Too many recommendations made by the review panel may be unachievable • Requires resources to provide education and training to staff in order for changes to be implemented.

(Adapted from Bull and Veall 2009, Rogers 2006 and Halligan et al. 2002)

Lewin's Force-Field Analysis model of change

Lewin (Sale 2005) discusses using a Force-Field Analysis (figure 4.6) and describes the notion of examining the forces at work and manipulating any or

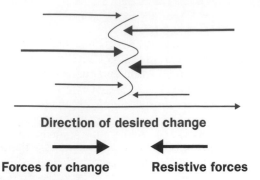

Direction of desired change

Forces for change   **Resistive forces**

Figure 4.6 Lewin's Force-Field Analysis model. (Lewin 1953, cited in Sale 2005)

all of these forces to achieve change. In order for this analysis to work, there needs to be a movement in thinking. Lewin describes this as taking place over three stages:

1. Unfreezing
2. Change
3. Refreezing.

Unfreezing

During the unfreezing stage, participants in the process will acknowledge that change is necessary and that current systems/processes require changing. The proposed changes may include an assessment of the current situation, for example a change in

* the organization
* management
* practice.

Once assessment has taken place, an action plan will be instigated.

Change

The acknowledgement that change is required will enable the use of a Force-Field Analysis during the change stage of Lewin's model. This analysis can take place only if unfreezing occurs. The Force-Field Analysis shows how change can be aided by reducing resistive forces effectively while progressively increasing the driving forces (Swage 2004). The resisting and driving forces are identified by each arrow; and if the thickness of the arrows varies, this will highlight the strength of the resistor or driver; the thicker the arrow the stronger the force.

Refreezing

Refreezing occurs when the action plan has been implemented, the changes in practice become the norm and the quality of care improved because the drivers have been strengthened and the resistors weakened.

Worked example from practice: medication errors

If we return to the worked example using Ishikawa's fishbone analysis of medication errors discussed in chapter 3 (figure 3.2), we can see a number of causes identified by the team that could be used to explain the reasons leading to medication errors.

In order to facilitate any change and improvement in quality care, the next stage for the team could be to use their initial analysis and identify the key drivers and resistors linked to medication errors; the beginning of this analysis can be seen in figure 4.7.

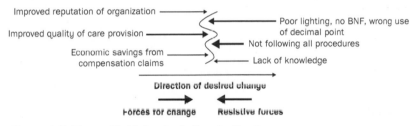

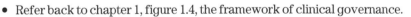

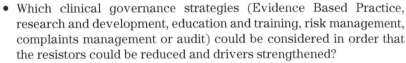

Figure 4.7 Force-Field Analysis for medication errors.

Having added the thick and thin arrows (drivers and resistors); the next stage for the team will be to consider which clinical governance strategies could be used to reduce the resistors and strengthen the drivers.

Activity

- Refer back to chapter 1, figure 1.4, the framework of clinical governance.
- Which clinical governance strategies (Evidence Based Practice, research and development, education and training, risk management, complaints management or audit) could be considered in order that the resistors could be reduced and drivers strengthened?

You may have considered risk management because of the poor lighting, no BNF, and wrong use of decimal point. You may also have considered education and training due to the lack of knowledge and finally, audit to mea-

Table 4.3 Critique of Lewin's Force-Field Analysis model

Strengths	Limitations
• It is a simple tool. • It is easy to understand and use. • Helps teams identify the strengths of resistors and drivers of change. • Helps teams to prioritize resistors and drivers through the thickness of arrows.	• It is only part of Lewin's wider Planned Approach to Change, and is therefore somewhat simplistic; as discussed in further detail below.

sure the change in practice and reduction of medication errors and financial compensation costs. These clinical governance strategies will be discussed in chapters 5 and 6.

Table 4.3 identifies some of the strengths and limitations of Lewin's model of change.

The four A's model of change

Barrett (2003), focusing on change in a healthcare setting, discussed a four staged process of change, whether macro or micro, which he identified as the four A's of change:

1. Antecedence
2. Analysis of options
3. Action on change
4. Aftermath of change.

Stage 1: Antecedence

This part of the process involves identifying the need for change, and Barrett (2003) suggests the following seven prompts:

1. Awakening – realizing that there are challenges to the status quo
2. Reactionary – includes an increase in patient/user complaints
3. Imposition hierarchy – top-down imposed change
4. Inverted hierarchy – bottom-up request for change
5. Maturation – evolution of the individual or organization
6. Adaptation – changes to procedures or processes
7. Invention – keeping abreast of changes in technology, drugs, surgical techniques, and so on.

Antecedence is key to the process of change, as opposition to change will be reduced if there is an understanding of why change is required. Barrett (2003) suggests that situational analysis is an important part of antecedence as it looks at the current situation. He suggests the use of two simple tools, SWOT (Mullins 2010) and PESTLE (Mullins 2010), which are discussed in greater detail in chapter 3.

Stage 2: Analysis of options

The next stage in the process is a considered analysis of options and the communication of these to the decision-makers involved in the change process. For this to take place effectively there needs to be an 'intention to act' (Barett 2003:154). Having choice, that is, a number of options, can result in uncertainty and decision-makers need to be aware of this and be able to cope with possible dilemmas in order to achieve the desired change. There is an extensive literature concerning decision-making, but this will not be discussed here.

Stage 3: Action on change

Identifying problem areas and opportunities for change is often the remit of one or more individuals whom Barrett (2003) refers to as change agents (from Broome 1998:87): 'Someone who identifies major problem areas, identifies the opportunities for change, builds readiness and commitment, builds a renewing system through creating a climate for change and establishes internal capacity to sustain the change effort, evaluate it and review it.'

A change agent may be internal or external to an organization, depending on the required change, and must motivate and deal with conflict as the proposed change is being discharged. Cahill (1995) describes three types of change agent:

1. Adopters hear about successful change and incorporate it into their practice (note the synergy with Roger's (1983) term in his Classification of Adopters, previously discussed).
2. Generators motivate and change attitudes.
3. Implementers initiate change once a decision to change has been recognized by generators.

It is widely agreed that, in order to implement change, a theoretical approach needs to be taken and many would use Lewin's three-step change at this stage of the process. This is the case in the article by Barrett (2003) where the three-step model has been used simplistically and in isolation.

It is widely believed that Lewin's three -step model is his key contribution to organizational change, but Burnes (2004) argues that Lewin did not intend this model to be used in isolation. What often seems to be forgotten is that Lewin was a humanitarian and his work stemmed from a passion to resolve social conflict, particularly the problems associated with minority or disadvantaged groups. He believed that using a Planned Approach to Change, which includes Field Theory, Group Dynamics and Action Research together with the three-step model could bring about change at an individual, group, organizational and societal level (Burnes 2004). What seems to have happened is that theorists have unpicked Lewin's Planned Approach to Change, merely focusing on the three-step model. This is highlighted by Hendry (1996:624) who stated, 'Scratch any account of creating and managing a change and the idea that change is a three-stage process which necessarily begins with a process of unfreezing will not be far below the surface.' This said, Barrett (2003) does recommend using Lewin's three-step theory as a theoretical approach to change but also calls for the identification of change strategies, focusing on three general strategies:

1. Rational-empirical strategy: This is based on the premise that many are guided by self-interest and reason and if they see the proposed change as benefitting them, they will support it. This is normally a top-down approach.
2. Power-coercive strategy: Also a top-down approach where those in authority instruct others to change.
3. Normative-reductive strategy: This is a bottom-up approach to change and is values led. Values and perceptions are altered and new norms are formed.

Strategies 1 and 2 may be used where compliance with legal directives is required, for example health and safety legislation, whereas strategy 3 is more appropriate for bringing about social change that benefits all stakeholders, for example patients, carers and staff.

Whichever of the above strategies is used, the change agent needs to demonstrate good *leadership* skills. Leaders may be either emergent (the leader is either informally chosen or formally elected by members of the group) or imposed (the leader is appointed or elected by a person or group external to the team to be led) (Sanchez-Cortes 2012) and may adopt one of three leadership styles (Mullins 2010):

1. Autocratic
2. Democratic
3. Laissez-faire.

Tannenbaum and Schmidt (1973, cited in Mullins 2010) presented a leadership continuum in which leaders may change their style to suit the situation. The categories of leadership in this continuum go from dictatorial to autocratic to democratic to laissez-faire.

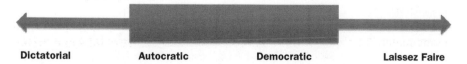

Dictatorial   Autocratic   Democratic   Laissez Faire

Dictatorial and laissez-faire are extremes in style, with a dictatorial leader making decisions without consultation and the latter unable to make quick and significant decisions.

Democratic leadership (Mullins 2010) is participative and promotes motivation, productivity and cohesiveness and in most change situations would be the leadership style of choice. However, it must be recognized that a democratic form of leadership would not be appropriate in an emergency situation, for example the leadership style required by a nurse co-ordinating the resuscitation of a patient. Here a dictatorial style would be required.

An integral part of good leadership is the ability to *motivate*, and there is a plethora of literature on motivation, with early work being undertaken by Maslow (1954), McClelland (1961), Vroom (1964). All agree that communication is key to motivation, and this is endorsed by Marquis and Huston (1998) who show how leaders use communication to motivate staff to embrace change.

Implementing change is essential to Barrett's process and preparation and planning play key roles at this stage. Resistance to change is also natural, but, if managed well, can lead to group cohesion and good group decisions. Gillies (1994) gives five suggestions to resolving conflict:

1. Competition and power
2. Smoothing
3. Avoidance
4 Compromise
5. Collaboration.

With the fifth option being the most suitable in managing change. A collaborative approach to decision-making would involve recognition that conflict exists, confronting the issues and collaboratively trying to resolve the issues whilst including all stakeholders in the process.

Stage 4: Aftermath of change

Whatever the change, Barrett (2003) suggests that a *contingency plan* needs to be in place, which allows a return to the pre-change position if, for whatever reason, the proposed change is unsuccessful. This supports the notion of a trial period of change with the ability to return to the pre-change position if necessary, thus reducing the possibility of fear of failure and risk. And finally, the process must be *evaluated*.

To conclude, Barrett (2003) posits that a structured process needs to be in place in order to implement a successful change and that his four A's provides such. However, there are still some strengths and limitations to this model (table 4.4).

We have considered four models that teams could use to facilitate the management of change and each of these models has strengths and limitations.

Table 4.4 Critique of Barrett's four A's model of change

Strengths	Limitations
• Sets out a process for change management, offering four clear steps • Another 'bottom-up' model • Engages service users and staff in quality improvement programmes • Motivates staff to continually develop the quality of healthcare provision by offering a fallback position (contingency plan).	It uses Lewin's three-step change theory and therefore is somewhat simplistic (as discussed above).

Activity

- Reflect on your own practice.
- Take each model in turn and decide whether you like or dislike the model (Diffusion of Innovation, RAID, Lewin's Force-Field Analysis and four A's).
- What is your rationale for these decisions?
- Can you identify any other strengths and limitations?
- Choose your preferred model.
- Consider an area of practice where the quality of care could be improved.
- Consider how you could apply your preferred model to your practice.

Key point summary

In order to improve the quality of care provided within healthcare, managing change and innovation needs to be a constant process. Resistance and uncertainty linked to change and innovation can be expected and therefore a transition phase is important. It is not possible to change everything at one time and so if the drivers and resistors are identified, healthcare professionals will be able to prioritize the changes and these can be addressed incrementally.

- It is the healthcare professional's responsibility to raise concerns about quality of care, although this may have repercussions.
- Change needs to be collaborative, that is, patients, carers and staff should be involved in a decision to change and in the change management process.
- Change needs to follow a process.
- A number of change management models can be utilized to drive the change initiative.

Implications for practice

- Any one of the four models for change may be used to facilitate change in a healthcare setting. All have strengths and limitations and these need to be taken into consideration when adopting a model.
- With an understanding of the Diffusion of Innovations model, if you are an early adopter remember to support team members who are either late adopters or laggards.
- Change takes time and therefore needs to be supported by management adopting appropriate leadership styles.

End-of-chapter questions

- What are the main barriers to change?
- Why does change need to be collaborative?
- How do developmental, transitional and transformational change differ?

See the Appendix on page 192 for suggested answers to these questions.

References

Attree M (2007) Factors influencing nurses' decisions to raise concerns about care quality. *Journal of Nursing Management*, 15 (4), 392–402

Barr J and Dowding L (2012) *Leadership in health care.* London: Sage

Barrett G (2003) How to manage change: The four A's of change. *Journal of Neonatal Nursing*, 9 (5), 153–157 (reader pages R84–R89)

Beerel A (2009) *Leadership and change management.* London: Sage

Bishop S (2010) *Develop your assertiveness.* London: Kogan Page

Broome A (1998) *Managing change: Essentials of nursing management* (2nd ed.). London: Macmillan

Bull K and Veall A (2009) Developing a diabetes link-nurse programme using the RAID quality improvement model. *Journal of Diabetes Nursing*, 13 (8), 298–304

Burnes B (2004) Kurt Lewin and the planned approach to change: A re-appraisal. *Journal of Management Studies*, 4, 977–1002

Cahill J (1995) Innovation and the role of the change agent. *Professional Nurse*, 11 (1), 57–58

Carnall C (2007) *Managing change in organisations.* London: Prentice Hall

Chambers R, Boath E and Rogers D (2007) *Clinical effectiveness and clinical governance made easy* (4th ed.). Oxford: Radcliffe

Gillies DA (1994) *Nursing management: A systems approach* (3rd ed.). London: WB Sauders

Gottwald M and Goodman-Brown J (2012) *A guide to practical health promotion.* Maidenhead: Open University Press

Halligan A, Wall D and O'Neill S (2002) Clinical governance: Sharing practical experiences – developing a national clinical governance resource. *British Journal of Clinical Governance*, 7 (1), 53–56

Haxby E, Hunter, DH and Jaggar S (2010) *An introduction to clinical governance and patient safety.* New York: Oxford University Press

Hendry C (1996) Understanding and creating whole orgnanizational change through learning theory. *Human Relations,* 48 (5), 621–641

Hopson B, Sacally M and Stafford K (2000) *Transitions: The challenge of change.* Chalford: Management Books

Iles V and Sutherland K (2001) *Organisational change: A review for healthcare managers, professionals and researchers.* London: London School of Hygiene and Tropical Medicine

Jackson D, Peters K, Andrew S, Edenborough M, Halcomb E, Luck L, Salamson Y and Wilkes L (2010) Understanding whistle-blowing: Qualitative insights from nurse whistle-blowers. *Journal of Advanced Nursing,* 66 (10), 2194–2201

Kotter J and Schlesinger L (2008) Choosing strategies for change. *Harvard Business Review,* July–Aug., 1–11

Kubler Ross E (1969) *On death and dying.* New York: Macmillan

Lewin K (1951) *Field theory in social science.* New York: Harper and Row

McClelland D (1961) *The Achieving Society.* New York: Van Nostrand Reinhold

McSherry R and Pearce P (2002) *Clinical governance: A guide to implementation for healthcare professionals.* Oxford: Blackwell

Marquis BL and Huston CJ (1998) *Management decision-making for nurses: 124 case studies* (3rd ed.). Philadelphia: Lippincott

Maslow A (1954) *Motivation and Personality.* New York: Harper and Row

Morrison V and Bennett P (2006) *An introduction to health psychology.* London: Prentice Hall

Mullins L (2010) *Management and organisational behaviour* (9th ed.). London: Prentice Hall

Naidoo J and Wills J (2009) *Foundations for health promotion.* London: Bailliere Tindall Elsevier

Nutbeam D and Harris E (2004) *Theory in a nutshell.* London: McGraw-Hill

Parkin P (2009) *Managing change in healthcare: Using action research.* London: Sage

Rogers E (1983) *Diffusion of innovations.* New York: Free Press

Rogers P (2006) RAID methodology: The NHS clinical governance team's approach to service improvement. *Clinical Governance: An International Journal* 11, (1), 69–80

Sale D (2005) *Understanding clinical governance and quality assurance: Making it happen.* Basingstoke: Palgrave Macmillan

Sanchez-Cortes D, Aran O, Mast MS and Gatica-Perez D (2012) A non-verbal behaviour approach to identify emergent leaders in small groups. *Multimedia,* 14 (3), 816–832

Sullivan E and Garland G (2013) *Practical leadership and management in healthcare: For nurses and allied health professionals.* London: Pearson

Swage T (2004) *Clinical governance in healthcare practice.* Oxford: Butterworth Heinemann

Tannenbaum R and Schmidt WH (1973) *How to choose a leadership pattern. Harvard Business Review,* 51 (3), 162–180

Vroom VH (1964) *Work and Motivation.* New York: Wiley

5

Implementing clinical governance strategies through education and training

Mary Gottwald

Chapter contents

- Learning objectives
- Introduction
- Learning
- Lifelong learning
- Continuing professional development
- Individual, team and organizational levels of education and training
- Identifying individual learning needs
- Linking learning needs and personal development reviews
- Learning organizations
- Organizational culture
- Worked examples of education and training
- Key point summary
- Implications for practice
- End-of-chapter questions
- References

Learning objectives

By the end of this chapter the reader will be better able to

- consolidate understanding of lifelong learning and continuing professional development

- identify a variety of methods that could be used to facilitate learning at all levels, through education and training
- understand how education and training impact on the culture of organization.

Introduction

The focus of this chapter is on education and training – one of the key clinical governance strategies. Clinical governance and continuous quality improvement (CQI) can be successful only if healthcare organizations value their staff by having education and training structures in place. These structures are essential to empower clinical and non-clinical staff to engage in education and training.

Concepts of lifelong learning and continuing professional development will be explored as well as the need for cultural change within health and social care organizations. VARK will be discussed as a means to understanding one's own learning style and practical suggestions on how education and training must be included at the individual, team and organizational level, will be considered. The chapter will conclude with a discussion on organizational culture, by making links to education and training.

Learning

There is a plethora of literature published in relation to learning, for example Bandura, Maslow, Piaget, Kolb, Dewey, Honey and Mumford, Skinner and Pavlov. However, it is not the remit of this chapter to discuss these theorists, and readers with an interest are advised to explore this literature independently.

Learning is a broad concept and comprises changes to knowledge, skills, attitudes and behaviour; it can be both formal and informal. In order to continuously update the evidence base of our practice and provide safe quality healthcare, learning must be lifelong and therefore ultimately this involves change (Mullins 2010). Learning ought to be a feature of organizational culture in healthcare organizations, and strategies for CPD staff development should be a part of any organization's business plans (Gopee and Galloway 2009).

Formal learning

The learning takes place in the classroom, is assessed and qualifications may be awarded.

Informal learning

Learning can also be informal, opportunistic and experiential in that it occurs through observation within a social context and healthcare practice environment. An example of opportunistic learning is professional socialization (Brennan and McSherry 2006, Brown et al. 2013).

Professional socialization

Professional socialization can be defined as 'a process whereby a person gains the knowledge, skills and identity that are characteristic of a professional and is a developmental process of adult socialization' (Becker Hentz 2005 cited in Brown et al. 2013:555).

In their research, Brennan and McSherry (2006) explore the transitional process and professional socialization from healthcare assistant to student nurse. It can be extrapolated therefore that the same process will occur throughout pre-registration programmes. Healthcare students experience a transitional process whereby their behaviour changes in relation to their identity, occupational roles and relationships and consequently they become 'professionally socialized' into their specific profession. This also involves taking on board the profession's values and norms which are not necessarily teachable.

Professional socialization may include

1. Culture shock
2. Anticipated socialization.

Culture shock

Students may experience confusion in relation to understanding their occupational role identity, which could lead to role conflict and role ambiguity, and hence some students may take longer to socialize into their profession (Brown et al. 2013). Brennan and McSherry (2006) identify this confusion as experiencing a 'culture shock'. Not only do they have to learn about the theory underpinning practice but also about professional aspects such as accountability, professional responsibility and professional and ethical codes of conduct. This culture shock may then become 'transition shock' as nursing students move into their first role of newly graduated nurses (Duchscher 2009). This may occur as new nursing professionals need to immerse themselves into potentially stressful and intense professional practice.

Anticipated socialization

Prior work experience whilst at school may have included working in a nursing home or rehabilitation ward, and as a result of this experience students may enter their pre-registration programme with ideas about the values of their profession and have a comfortable feeling when working within healthcare. Brown et al. (2013:565) suggest this is 'anticipated socialization'.

However, pre-registration placements could include working in other more challenging areas such as psychiatric units, prisons or specialized burns units, and so students will need to go through a transitional period adapting and developing their knowledge and skills to enable them to work in these varied areas of practice, some of which could be challenging. Pre-registration students who have undertaken prior work experience will have gained knowledge as well as practical experience and consequently could be considered to be at an advantage. However, transferring this to different settings and adapting may take time; therefore professional socialization can be challenging for everyone.

Lifelong learning

On graduation, pre-registration students are deemed to have achieved professional socialization. However, this should not be the end of their learning journey, and, as already stated, lifelong learning is imperative if organizations are constantly going to to improve the quality of healthcare provision. 'Lifelong learning depends on every health organization developing its learning environment' (Swage 2004:180) into one that is conducive to learning. Lifelong learning involves 'Changes and learning that continue throughout life, and takes places in a variety of ways and range of situations' (Mullins 2010:172).

It is therefore vital that healthcare organizations become learning organizations. This will be discussed in more detail towards the end of this chapter in the discussion on organizational culture.

Continuing professional development

Lifelong learning includes continuing professional development (CPD). The UK Royal College of Nursing (2007:2) state that 'Continuing Professional Development (CPD) is fundamental to the development of all health and social care practitioners, and is the mechanism through which high quality patient and client care is identified, maintained and developed.'

Self-development therefore is very much part of CPD and today keeping a portfolio and practising for a minimum number of hours is a compulsory requirement in order to maintain registration for many healthcare professions. The reason for this is because practitioners need to demonstrate that they are continually learning and updating their practice. Table 5.1 considers a number of CPD definitions and identifies some strengths and limitations.

One of the advantages of the Wright and Hill (2003) and Swage (2004) definitions is that the focus is on *both* the individual and the organization. Education and training related to the individual and organizational levels will be considered later on in this chapter.

Aims of continuing professional development (CPD)

There are two key aims of CPD (Swage 2004):

1. To make sure that healthcare professionals are provided with opportunities to develop their attributes, knowledge and skills, so they are enabled to progress along their career pathway. This then impacts on the second aim.
2. To make sure services continue to develop and provide an improved patient experience.

Table 5.1 Definitions of CPD

	Definition	Critique
Wright and Hill (2003:85)	'A purposeful, systematic activity by individuals and possibly their organizations, to maintain and develop the knowledge, skills and attributes which are needed for effective professional practice'.	Includes both the individual and organization. Focus is wider than just knowledge.
Swage (2004:6)	CPD programs are 'aimed at meeting the development needs of individual health professionals and the service needs of the organization are in place and supported locally and regularly monitored'.	Includes both the individual and organization. Focus on regular evaluation.
Mullins (2010:824)	'The process of planned, continuing development of individuals throughout their career'.	Does not consider the need of the organization.
Swage (2004:318)	'An individual taking responsibility for the development of his/her own career by systematically analysing development needs, identifying and using appropriate methods to meet these needs and regularly reviewing achievement compared against personal and career objectives'.	Does not consider the need of the organization. Focus on regular review and monitoring of objectives.

Figure 5.1 exemplifies how the aims of CPD can be illustrated by a continuous cycle of events. It also depicts how CPD is linked with appraisal.

Individual, team and organizational levels of education and training

In order to improve the quality of care provided and to ensure standards are met, clinicians need to ensure that they have up-to-date skills and knowledge and, as discussed in chapters 1 and 7, must make sure their practice is evidence-based. Links to clinical governance therefore need to be made between clinical effectiveness, research and development of practice. Organizations have to make certain that staff employed have the right attributes as well as skills and knowledge. However, the responsibility does not solely

Assessment of individual's needs
Assessment of organization's needs

Evaluation of the CPD process
Evaluation of benefits to the individual, patient and organization

Agreement of Personal Development Plans (PDP) / Personal Development Reviews (PDR) with ALL staff

Identification of training and education needs
Implementation of agreed objectives

Figure 5.1 CPD cycle. (Adapted from Sale 2005:96)

lie with the organization and Sale (2005) suggests that education and training should occur at three levels. Figure 5.2 illustrates some educational activities that can be carried out at each of these levels.

1. Individual level
2. Team level
3. Organizational level.

INDIVIDUAL LEVEL

- Engage in short courses, e-learning, distance learning (Massive Online Open Courses), postgraduate courses.
- Reflective diaries.
- Use time outside of work.

TEAM LEVEL

- Multidisciplinary teams
- Workshops
- Seminars/lectures/tutorials
- Critical incidents
- Case studies
- Journal clubs
- Simulations

EDUCATION AND TRAINING

ORGANIZATIONAL LEVEL

- Induction/preceptorship programmes
- Provision of resources
- Provision of mandatory training

Figure 5.2 Levels of education and training. (Adapted from Wright and Hill 2003, Sale 2005)

Individual level

As discussed in chapter 1, practitioners are accountable and therefore responsible for making sure their practice is evidence-based. This also links to *effectiveness*, one of Maxwell's six dimensions of quality discussed in chapter 3. However, finances within health and social care organizations are limited and therefore individuals may well need to use some of their personal time as well as finances outside work to develop their knowledge.

Individuals must make sure they engage with and complete all mandatory training and they could also utilize opportunities to engage in e-learning/online distance learning/Massive Online Open Courses (MOOCS), short courses (both accredited and non-accredited), postgraduate certificates, diplomas or Masters programmes. They could access the organization's Learning and Development Centre to identify relevant training opportunities delivered within the organization.

Individuals could also undertake a *SWOT analysis* as discussed in chapter 3. Once reflection on their strengths, weakness, opportunities and threats has occurred, further learning can be facilitated through setting mutually agreed objectives and action plans linked to the SWOT analysis. These objectives would need to be agreed with their line manager. Individuals need to engage with agreed objectives, and reviewing these objectives at their next annual personal development review (PDR, appraisal). It is also useful to have an interim review to check progress and to see if further support is needed from line managers so that action plans are achieved (Wright and Hill 2003, Sale 2005).

Activity

- Consider your own area of practice.
- What recent education and training have you undertaken at the individual level?

For a wider understanding on Department of Health plans access the following link: http://www.gov.uk Education outcomes framework (DoH 2013) for healthcare workforce.

The Department of Health (2012:4) published 'liberating the NHS: Developing the Healthcare Workforce: from Design to Delivery'. The Education Outcomes Framework (EOF) included in this document aims to make sure that staff 'have the right skills, behaviours and training, available in the right numbers, to support the delivery of excellent healthcare and health improvement'.

Identifying individual learning needs

There are a number of methods that are used to identify individual learning needs. This chapter will consider VARK.

VARK

VARK is a short questionnaire that Fleming devised in 1987. It is accessible in a variety of languages and is quick to complete online as it has only 16 questions. Fleming stresses that VARK is not a learning style inventory as such because it looks at one aspect only. It does not consider dimensions such as *when* individuals like to learn or *what* makes them motivated (makes them engage in small group work, one to one tutorials). Despite this, it is still useful and can be used by individuals to help them further understand how they learn best. It could also be used within teams to help understand individual differences and build relationships; however, adhering to the copyright regulations is essential.

> ### Activity
>
> - Access the VARK website http://www.vark-learn.com/english and complete the questionnaire.
> - Once you have identified your preference(s), access the help sheets, which will provide strategies to facilitate your learning.

Once you have completed the VARK questionnaire, you will have identified your learning preferences and these are shown in table 5.2.

Table 5.2 Dimensions of VARK

Visual	Individuals with this preference like to learn from graphs, mind maps, histograms, that is, any symbolic or graphic form.
Auditory	Listening to oral presentations is preferred and these individuals also like to engage and interact with lectures, seminars, discussion groups.
Read/write	Diaries, lists, bullet points, handouts, leaflets are preferred methods of learning.
Kinaesthetic	Here learning takes place through all senses and these individuals like to learn through concrete examples and in particular like to be able to link these examples to their own experience.

We have considered a variety of methods that could be used to facilitate learning at the individual level. The next activity will help you to link your learning preferences to methods of learning.

> **Activity**
>
> * Having identified your learning preferences, consider which methods suit you best.
> * Do practical simulations and workshops, lectures, online learning opportunities, case study or journal club discussions suit your learning preferences?
> * Which of the strategies identified in VARK could facilitate your learning further?

Linking learning needs and personal development reviews

The flow diagram (figure 5.3) below illustrates four steps that could help you to prepare for your next personal development review (PDR) / personal development plan (PDP).

Writing objectives

When writing objectives, they need to be SMART (Mullins 2010):

* Specific
* Measurable
* Achievable
* Realistic/relevant
* Timeframe/time bound.

If each objective contains all of the above elements, it is much easier to evaluate and measure them. For example:

1. By the end of 2014, I will submit an article to a peer reviewed journal.
2. By the end of July 2015, I will have read at least one journal article per month.

> **Activity**
>
> * Consider these objectives.
> * Are they SMART? If so, why? If not, why not?
> * Does your team set SMART Objectives?

Step 1:

Step 2:

Step 3:

Step 4:

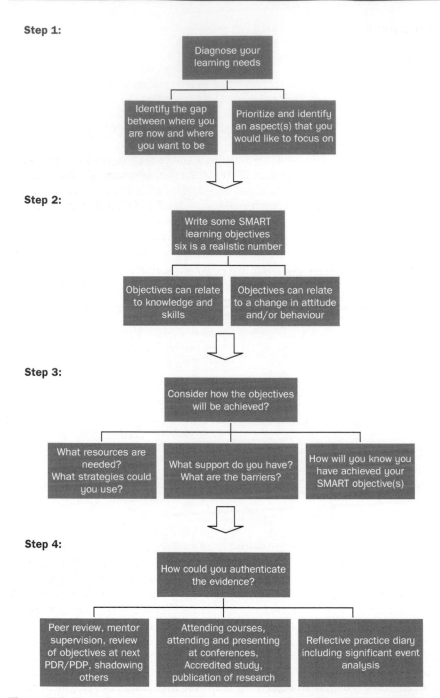

Figure 5.3 Identifying learning development. (Adapted from Swage 2004:181)

Team level

Education and training at this level probably works best if delivered to multidisciplinary teams, as this fosters better communication and collaboration and understanding of roles. One advantage of learning in teams is that members tend to have the shared value 'to meet the needs of their patients' (Wright and Hill 2003:168). Further education and training may be one of the requirements following a 'near miss' event or a complaint, to ensure that the mistake does not happen again.

A variety of methods could be used to facilitate learning at the team level. For example, small group work could be organized, in which case studies and/ or critical incidents are discussed and action plans agreed. Journal clubs could be established, in which all members agree to read and discuss one paper per month in small groups, alternatively members could take it in turns to agree to read and present key points from one current journal paper. This may reduce the pressure with regard to time. Workshops could be organized using manikins, and actors could be employed to role play and discuss scenarios.

All of these discussions encourage reflective practice and facilitate understanding of current practice and the evidence base for this. Learning can also be shared in everyday practice through peer observation and demonstration and through mentoring undergraduates, new graduates and healthcare assistants (Sale 2005).

Activity

- Consider your own area of practice.
- What education and training is provided at the team level?
- Have you been provided with recent opportunities to engage in further learning at the team level?

Organizational level

On employment all health and social care staff can expect structures to be provided that include an induction/preceptorship, mentoring programme. They can also expect the organization to provide continuous clinical supervision. In the context of clinical governance, the induction should also include learning activities so that staff can understand the clinical governance framework; how this framework links to the organization's strategic directives as well as government directives and their role in ensuring clinical governance strategies are implemented. In order for education and training to be successful the organization needs to provide resources, both in terms of finances and time, so that development objectives identified in personal development plans (PDPs) can be achieved. Resources also need to be provided to enable mandatory training to be completed, for example health and safety, infection and prevention procedures, moving and handling, resuscitation. Nowadays, some of this mandatory training takes place through e-learning.

One of the advantages of e-learning is that staff can learn at a time that suits them. However, organizations must still allow dedicated time for this learning and staff need to manage their time to ensure this learning takes place. E-learning may include online learning that organizations have developed and so is accessible only to employees of that organization. It may also include courses provided by universities that are open only to those registered on specific programmes. E-learning may also include courses known as MOOCs. Since 2007 there has been a move for institutions to provide opportunities for learners to engage in Massive Open Online Courses (MOOCS). MOOCs originated in Canada and up to a point are free of charge. They provide opportunities for those interested in learning to engage in flexible, open access, non-credited courses accessed via the web. Anyone throughout the world with a desire to develop their learning can register. Although non-credited, assessments are included and on successful completion of the course, certificates are provided. One of the advantages of MOOCs is that individuals can liaise across the world, sharing ideas and experiences (Daniel 2012).

Activity

- Consider your own area of practice.
- What education and training is provided at the organizational level?
- Have you been provided with recent opportunities to engage in further learning at the organizational level?

Learning organizations

We have discussed the importance of learning occurring at the individual, team and organizational level. An organization in which learning is fostered is known as a *learning organization*. This type of organization continually provides opportunities for employees to develop their knowledge and skills in order to provide excellent quality care. A learning organization is one that 'encourages and facilitates the learning and development of people at all levels of the organization, values the learning and simultaneously transforms itself' (Mullins 2010:827), so that it becomes 'an efficient adaptive unit' (Wright and Hill 2003:193).

Characteristics of a learning organization

There are a number of characteristics that identify whether an organization is a learning organization or not (Reineck 2002, Barr and Dowding 2012, Mullins 2010):

1. Staff feel that what they do is important, and valued (see Schein's middle level of organizational culture *values and beliefs*, discussed below). If staff feel valued and therefore more motivated, staff retention will be high.
2. Staff are continually provided with opportunities to develop their knowledge and skills in relation to patient care. They are encouraged to try different approaches. They are also encouraged and facilitated to gain an understanding on how the different levels of the organization function.
3. Staff are encouraged to evaluate interventions and explore the strengths and limitations of these interventions.
4. There is mutual respect amongst employees and staff as different grades work together as colleagues, supporting each other in their learning (see Schein's inner layer of organizational culture *underlying assumptions*, discussed below).
5. There is a shared vision within teams.
6. Communication is good at all levels.

Activity

- Reflect on the examples of poor quality care given in chapter 1 (figures 1.1 and 1.2).
- Do you think these were learning organizations? If not, why not?

Gopee and Galloway (2009) suggest that a positive organizational culture of an organization can impact on the likelihood of that organization becoming a learning organization.

Organizational culture

For staff to be able to engage in lifelong learning and CPD, the culture of organization needs to support learning. Culture is 'something that is shared by members of an organisation . . . the glue that holds together potentially diverse individuals' (Kelemen 2005:128). Mullins (2010:739) defines it as 'how things are done around here', in other words, what behaviour is acceptable and what behaviour is unacceptable. Huczynski and Buchanan (2007:623) provide us with a more in-depth definition: 'Culture is the collection of relatively uniform and enduring values, beliefs, customs, traditions and practices that are shared by an organization's members, learned by new recruits, and transmitted from one generation of employees to the next.'

This definition closely links to Schein's (2010) levels of culture, which will be discussed below. Clinical governance is about changing organizational culture in a systematic and demonstrable way, moving away from a culture of blame to one of learning, so that quality infuses all aspects of the organization's work (Department of Health 1998). However, organizational culture is not tangible and is hard to measure (Carnall 2007).

Models of culture

There are a number of models of organizational culture, such as Schein's (2010) and Handy's (1999), and Johnson's (1988) cultural web and Hofstede's (1968) characteristics of culture. This chapter will consider two:

1. Schein's levels of organizational culture
2. Handy's four types of culture.

Levels of organizational culture

If staff accept the traditions, values and beliefs held within the organization, then they are more likely to become motivated and inspired to learn, and therefore the organizational strategic objectives are more likely to be achieved.

Schein (2010) identifies three levels of organizational culture, which could be depicted by the three layers of an onion (figure 5.4).

1. Artefacts
2. Values and beliefs
3. Underlying assumptions.

Artefacts

This is the outer and most superficial layer of the onion. Schein (2010) states that artefacts within the organization are tangible. They can be seen by everyone whether employed or not, for example

- the furniture: the type of office furniture reflects certain privileges and grades

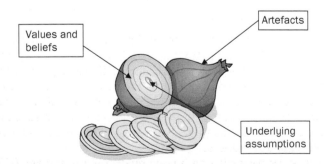

Figure 5.4 Layers of organizational culture.

- equipment
- logos used on headed notepaper, or on signs at entrances to hospitals or community centres
- uniforms that identify different staff (porters, nurses, doctors, allied health professionals, canteen staff).

Artefacts can also be heard and experienced, and include the behaviours that staff follow such as how staff speak to one another and display their emotions. In some organizations, this could be a bullying and blame culture, as discussed in chapter 2. If the culture within the organization is one of bullying and blame, this could impede learning. Artefacts also include other behavioural manifestations such as rituals, for example the hospital ward round.

Values and beliefs

These form the middle layer of the onion and are not visible. Schein (2010) goes on to suggest that individuals have their own notions on what is right and wrong. Organizational culture at this level will occur once the team agree and adopt shared beliefs, such as the importance of providing quality health-care or reporting adverse incidents, for example needle stick or medication errors.

This layer includes unwritten rules (norms) that tell employees how to behave in a wide variety of situations, for example not all health and social care professionals wear uniform, in particular in the community and mental health organizations. Yet there is an expectation that staff and students on placement will present themselves in a professional manner. If the beliefs and values of a team are different from those that support high performance, then the desired behaviour will not be reflected in the observed behaviour. Norms and values are linked. The norm of not displaying emotion whilst at work is linked to the value of self-discipline. Members of an organization that has a specific culture will hold values and conform to cultural norms, because their underlying assumptions support these values and norms.

Underlying assumptions

Underlying assumptions are at the deepest level, form the centre of the onion and are not visible. Schein (2010) suggests that these underlying assumptions form the core of an organization's culture. There may be an underlying assumption that experienced senior staff are respected and so students on clinical placement become 'socialized' to accept the cultural value of respecting senior staff. When a solution to a problem is continually successful, then the method is repeated. These then become unconscious behaviours that are accepted and taken for granted.

When staff work towards continuous quality improvement (CQI), there is a quality culture within the organization. Strong organizational cultures work towards achieving common goals and standards (total quality management – TQM) and strong organizational cultures reward and value staff, who in turn are more likely to become motivated and inspired to engage in lifelong learning and CPD activities. Chapter 6 will discuss these concepts in greater detail.

Cultural types

Handy (1999) considers four types of culture that can exist within organizations:

1. Power culture
2. Role culture
3. Task culture
4. Person culture.

Power culture

This can be depicted as a spider's web where centralized control is undertaken by one individual or a few key individuals. There are then 'rays of power and influence spreading out from the central figure' (Handy 1999:184) and the closer individuals are to the centre the greater the influence and power.

Role culture

Handy (1999) depicts this culture as a Greek temple. The pillars of this temple are independent departments such as the Human Resource Department, Learning and Development Centre, Finance Department, Physiotherapy Department, Accident and Emergency Department. These departments support the pediment at the top of the temple. Within each department staff are employed because they have the skills and attributes required for the job. Staff are given a contract which includes a job description that identifies their key roles and responsibilities. The pediment of this temple can be seen as the senior management who are responsible for co-ordinating all procedures.

Rewards tend to occur within this culture. Opportunities are provided for further staff development through education and training and this can lead to promotion within the organization. However, there are occasions when teams will come together to work on a specific task. In this situation there may be conflicts over leadership of this newly formed group and the security of role culture may be undermined.

Task culture

'Task culture is job or project orientated' (Handy 1999:187) and can be depicted as a grid with the power lying at the junctures. The focus of this culture is to ensure the job or project is completed and therefore the right people with the right skills are employed and are accountable for particular jobs or projects. Organizations must ensure that these individuals are provided with further CPD opportunities. Individuals identify with the strategic objectives or the organization and work together so that the job is completed.

Person culture

Handy (1999) depicts this culture as a constellation of stars. It is not likely that this culture solely appears in health and social care organizations, because person culture lacks structure and corporate objectives. As the structure is minimal, individuals are enabled to do their own thing more effectively. Each cultural type has strengths and limitations, some of which are identified in table 5.3.

Table 5.3 Critique of cultural types

	Strengths	Limitations
Power	Will respond quickly to incidents. Decisions are taken on the balance of influence. Decisions made by a few individuals.	Dependent on the capabilities of the key individuals at the centre. Continued success may depend on succession.
Role	Formal departments co-ordinated by senior management. Standardization occurs through common procedures. Rewards staff through promotion.	Due to the formality of role culture organizations may be slow to recognize the need to change and are slow to undertake change. Individuals who are accustomed to power can become disillusioned.
Task	Jobs and projects get completed by empowered teams. The right individuals are employed with the right knowledge and skills.	Relies on good collaboration and teamwork. Individuals may lack the skills that role cultures possess. Individual needs are less important than team needs.
Person	The individual is the focal point and their basic needs are adhered to.	Minimalistic structure. The organization is subservient to the individual where individuals do their own thing.

(Adapted from Handy 1999)

Activity

Consider your organization. Is there a predominant culture or is there a mix of cultures within your organization? Where does it fit in with Handy's (1999) descriptions of organizational culture (power, role, task or person culture)?

- Is the emphasis on getting the job done (task culture)?
- Do the demands come from the top without much concern for your welfare as a person (power culture)?
- Are employees involved in decision-making (role culture)?
- Are there support mechanisms for staff, for example to manage stress within the working environment (person culture)?
- How do you as an individual, relate to the culture in your organization?

Reflect on these questions and consider the rationale that supports your answers.

Worked examples of education and training

This book has considered a number of quality issues – pressure ulcers, medication errors, falls, Ventilator Associated Pneumonia, needle stick injuries, violence, bullying and aggression, and hospital acquired infections. Tables 5.4 to 5.10 identify some examples of education and training at each of the levels discussed above.

Table 5.4 Pressure ulcers

Individual level:
Ensure awareness of wound management policy and how to report 'near misses'.

Team level:
Mandatory training on Venous Thrombotic Embolisms to make sure pressure ulcers do not occur due to immobilization.
Education and training needs assessment of teams. If staff make an error due to lack of awareness, then education and training must be provided, for example lack of awareness of who is at risk of developing a pressure sore due to poor nutrition, and the importance of hydration in relation to pressure sores.
Regular audits will lead to education and training if the incidence of pressure ulcers increases. For example, ensuring staff know the specialist beds that should be used or the requirements to regularly turn and examine common areas of risk.
Increase staff awareness on operational processes to follow.

(continued)

Table 5.4 (*Continued*)

Organizational level:
The incidence of pressure ulcers is auditable and therefore teams need to be aware of this.
Ensure staff are aware of NICE guidelines (http://nice.org.uk) and European guidelines; for example: http://epuap.org/guidelines (pressure ulcers).

Table 5.5 Medication errors

Individual level:
To be aware of own professional responsibility and subsequent development in the safe administration of medications. To be aware of the trust policy on 'report medication errors'.

Team level:
Following a 'near miss' or medication error CPD is important to ensure that double checking or three checks and five rights (right drug to the right patient in the right dose by the right route at the right time) procedures are followed (ISMP 2007).
Workshop following a 'near miss' – use this as a learning opportunity for the team, so that it is not the 'last domino' who gets the blame.

Organizational level:
During induction all staff will be made aware of the procedural rules designed by the organization to follow the five rights. Organizations may consider adding three further rights (right reason, right drug formulation and right line attachment) (ISMP 2007).

Table 5.6 Falls

Individual level:
Regardless of lack of time, staff must remind each other to make sure the cot sides are put back up when required (e.g. patient may have post-surgery psychosis or mental health issues).

Team level:
Supporting the education of teams in use of risk assessment tools, for example the Morse Falls Risk Assessment.
Ensure staff are aware of the falls team and how to contact this team.
Remind staff of processes to follow after an incident or 'near miss'.

Organizational level:
Dissemination of communication guidelines to all staff, to raise awareness of local processes.

Table 5.7 Ventilator Associated Pneumonia

Individual level:
To ensure own professional development by being up to date on the management
of ventilated patients and risks associated with the development of complications
from mechanical ventilation, including VAP.

Team level:
Increasing staff awareness of the availability of care bundles (see NICE
guidelines for further details http://www.NICE.org.UK/guidance/index.
jsp?action=articleando=38047)

Organizational level:
During induction all staff will be made aware of policies and procedures in place
in ICUs, high-dependency units and specialized wards to support withdrawal
from mechanical ventilation and thereby a reduction in VAP.
Staff will also need to be made aware of the policies on how to reduce the risk
once extubated on the high dependency unit, ICU or specialized unit.

Table 5.8 Needle stick injuries

Individual level:
Own personal and professional responsibility to ensure up to date on needle stick
injury policy, including how to avoid and so minimize the risk and how to report
and what action is required if a needle stick injury occurs.

Team level:
Ward information provided on location of sharps bins.
Best practice would include regular training on the processes to follow in order to
prevent needle stick injuries.
Processes accessible so that if a needle stick injury happens, staff know what
process to follow.

Organizational level:
Supported by the Occupational Health Department.
During induction all staff will be made aware of processes and procedures in place
to support the prevention of injuries; reporting near misses or actual injuries.

Table 5.9 Violence, bullying and aggression

Individual level:
Organizational policy varies and therefore staff must make sure they are aware of
local policy. They also need to check to see if it includes policies to follow for
both verbal intimidation and physical aggression.

(continued)

Table 5.9 (Continued)

Team level:
Team updates on current prevention and management of violence, bullying and aggression (VBA).Practice in breakaway techniques.
Make sure staff are aware of how to access procedural documents.

Organizational level:
Mandatory training – prevention and management of violence, bullying and aggression programmes (VBA). Breakaway techniques.

Table 5.10 Hospital acquired infections

Individual level:
Own personal and professional responsibility to ensure up to date on needle stick injury policy, including how to avoid and so minimize the risk and how to report and what action is required if an injury occurs.
Undertake mandatory training in hand washing, non-touch technique (NTT), Clostridium difficile and MRSA.

Team level:
Infection and prevention control nurse will provide regular updates on incidence of HAIs within the organization and therefore support training, for example isolation management.

Organizational level:
Induction programmes to make staff aware of local policies and audit processes.

All of the methods mentioned have strengths and limitations and therefore learners need to think about their learning styles as this will help identify methods that most suit their needs. Table 5.11 begins to identify strengths and limitations. However, what has not been included in this table is the requirement to be aware of learners' individual learning preferences.

Activity

Whilst you can engage in formal CPD events at the three levels discussed above, personal reading still remains key to personal development. The following will give you further information on the quality issues discussed in chapter 2:

- The Wound Repair and Regeneration Journal or American Journal of Critical Care (pressure ulcers).
- The Journal of the American Medical Association (medication errors and Ventilator Associated Pneumonia).

- NICE (National Institute for Health and Care Excellence) guidelines, for example clinical guideline 21 (CG21) for falls, CG42 (VAB–Violence, aggression and bullying).
- Nursing Times (needle stick injuries).
- *The Journal of Mental Health* (VAB), search for articles that discuss strengths and limitations of de-escalation and breakaway techniques.
- National Service Frameworks, for example NSF: Children, Young People and Maternity Services (DoH 2004), NSF for Older People (DoH 2001), NSF Mental Health (DoH 1999). We have explored a number of methods that could be used to facilitate learning at a variety of levels. Table 5.11 highlights some of the strengths and limitations of these methods.
- http://www.hcswtoolkit.nes.scot.nhs.uk/Healthcare support workers toolkit RCN

Table 5.11 Critique of methods used within education and training

	Strengths	Limitations
Journal clubs	Up-to-date research papers that focus on current practice can be explored	Requires commitment and motivation from individuals to read, summarize key points and apply learning to practice
Simulations, for example use of manikins, actors, computer programmes	Interactive and engaging	Resource intensive
Critical incident reviews/ case study discussions	Current and relevant to teams; therefore stimulating and motivating	Need time for reflection and can therefore be time consuming
Lectures	Can be delivered to large numbers	Take time to prepare, and lecturer may not engage the audience
Workshops	Generally 'hands on' and interactive	Due to small numbers could be costly if need to be repeated
E-learning/ distance learning	Undertaken at a convenient time and at individual's own pace	If participants do not engage in online discussions and debates, then the learning process could be lonely, and limited learning may occur.
Private study	Undertaken at a convenient time and at individual's own pace	Requires motivation and commitment and good time management skills.

Activity

- Earlier activities asked you to consider methods that are used at the individual, team and organizational levels, which would facilitate learning.
- Can you think of other methods?
- Table 5.11 provides one strength and one limitation. Reflect on these methods and consider further strengths and limitations.

Table 5.12 provides useful links to some profession specific CPD opportunities that you might like to explore.

Table 5.12 Accessing CPD opportunities via the internet

http://www.rcn.org.uk/ development/learning/ learningzone	• This will take you to the UK Royal College of Nursing website 'Learning Zone'. • This is a useful website for healthcare assistants, assistant practitioners, student and registered nurses who work in different settings. • Explore the varied opportunities that you have to engage in online continuing professional development (CPD). • For example you might be interested in engaging in learning activities in relation to patient safety or in supporting people's nutritional needs (relevant for pressure ulcers). You might also like to explore the guidance and legislation provided in relation to violence in the workplace and bullying and harassment in the workplace (VAB).
http://www.cot.co.uk	• This will take you to the College of Occupational Therapy website. • Resources are provided that enable practitioners to engage in lifelong learning and CPD opportunities. • Resources include interactive e-learning, video and printable resources. • Members of the British Association of Occupational Therapists can access an Interactive Learning Opportunities Database (ILOD).
http://www.csp.prg.uk/ professional -union/ careers-development/ cpd	• This will take you to the Chartered Society of Physiotherapy. • CPD opportunities are provided through a championing CPD project that facilitates peer-to-peer support for CPD development of skills and knowledge in the workplace through Learning Champions.

Key point summary

Education and training underpin the implementation of clinical governance strategies. Education can be both formal and informal and in a learning organization should take place at the individual, team and organizational level.

* It is both a personal and organizational responsibility that members of staff at all levels are engaged in CPD.
* In order to be a learning organization all members of staff will benefit from an annual appraisal or PDR.
* In order to take part in appropriate CPD activities, it is important for staff to understand their learning styles.

Implications for practice

* A match of individual and organizational values might impact on the retention of staff.
* Experienced staff need to be aware that new members of staff coming into their team may experience transition shock.
* Clinical staff as autonomous practitioners have a personal responsibility to engage in CPD.

End-of-chapter questions

1. What are the key differences between Schein's (2010) levels of culture?
2. Which is the most inclusive of Handy's (1999) four cultural types?
3. What is the disadvantage of this cultural type?

See the Appendix on page 193 for suggested answers to these questions.

References

Barr J and Dowding L (2012) *Leadership in health care.* London: Sage

Becker Henz P (2005) Education and socialisation to the professional nursing role. In: Masters K (ed) *Role development in professional nursing practice.* Sudbury: Jones and Bartlett, 99–127

Brennan G and McSherry R (2006) Exploring the transition and professional socialisation from healthcare assistant to student nurse. *Nurse Education in Practice*, 7 (4), 206–214

Brown J, Stevens J and Kermonde S (2013) Measuring student nurse professional socialisation: The development and implementation of a new instrument. *Nurse Education Today*, 33 (6), 565–573

Carnall C (2007) *Managing change in organizations* (5th ed.). London: Prentice-Hall

Daniel J (2012) Making sense of MOOCs: Musings in a maze of myth, paradox and possibility. *Journal of Interactive Media in Education*, 18 (http://jime.open.ac.uk/2012018, accessed 22.10.2013)

Department of Health (1998) *A first class service: Quality in the new NHS*. London: Department of Health

Department of Health (1999) *National Service Framework of Mental Health*. Available at https://www.gov.uk/government/uploads/system/uploads/attachment_data/file/198051/National_Service_Framework_for_Mental_Health.pdf (accessed 28.01.2014)

Department of Health (2001) *National service framework for older people*. Available at https://www.gov.uk/government/uploads/system/uploads/attachment_data/file/198033/National_Service_Framework_tor_Older_People.pdf (accessed 28.01.2014)

Department of Health (2004) National service framework: Children, young people and maternity services. Available at http://www.nhs.uk/NHSEngland/AboutNHSservices/Documents/NSF%20children%20in%20hospitlalDH_4067251[1].pdf (accessed 28.01.2014)

Department of Health (2012) *Liberating the NHS: Developing the healthcare workforce. From design to delivery*. Available at https://www.gov.uk/government/uploads/system/uploads/attachment_data/file/216421/dh_132087.pdf (accessed 20.01.2014)

Department of Health (2013) *The education outcomes framework*. London: Department of Health. Available at https://www.gov.uk/government/uploads/system/uploads/attachment_data/file/175546/Education_outcomes_framework.pdf (accessed 28.01.2014)

Duchscher J (2009) Transition shock: The initial stage of role adaptation for newly graduated Registered Nurses. *Journal of Advanced Nursing*, 65 (5), 1103–1113

Fleming N. (1987) A guide to learning styles VARK. Available at http://www.vark-learn.com/english/index.asp (accessed 22.10.2013)

Gopee N and Galloway J (2009) *Leadership and management in healthcare*. London: Sage

Handy C (1999) *Understanding organisations*. London: Penguin

Hofstede G (1968) *Cultures consequences*. Harmondsworth. Penguin.

Huczynski A and Buchanan D (2007) *Organisational behavior*. Harlow: Prentice Hall

Institute for Safe Medication Practices (ISMP) (2007) http://www.ismp.org/Newsletters/acutecare/articles/20070125.asp (accessed 30.10.2013)

Johnson G (1988) Rethinking incrementalism. *Strategic Management Journal*, 9 (1), 75–91

Keleman M (2005) *Managing quality*. London: Sage

Mullins L (2010) *Management and organisational behaviour*. London: Prentice Hall

NICE guidelines http://guidance.nice.org.uk/CG/Published (accessed 22.10.2013)

Reineck C (2002) Leadership's guiding light, part 2: Create a learning organization. *Nursing Management*, 33 (10), 13–18

Royal College of Nursing (2007) *A joint statement on continuing professional development for health and social care practitioners*. London: Royal College of Nursing

Sale D (2005) *Understanding clinical governance and quality assurance: Making it happen.* Basingstoke: Palgrave Macmillan

Schein E H (2010) *Organisational culture and leadership* (4th ed.). San Francisco: Jossey-Bass

Swage T (2004) *Clinical governance in healthcare practice.* London: Butterworth Heinemann

Wright J and Hill P (2003) *Clinical governance.* London: Churchill Livingstone

6

How clinical governance can be supported through Evidence Based Practice

Gail E Lansdown

Chapter contents

Learning objectives

This chapter will enable the reader to have a better understanding of

- definitions of Evidence Based Practice (EBP) and Values Based Practice (VBP)

- the application of EBP to healthcare
- defining problems
- searching for information
- finding solutions
- EBP and Integrated Care Pathways and Care Bundles.

Introduction

The previous chapter focused on education and training. This chapter will focus on the importance of EBP and how this can be applied to clinical governance.

Definitions of EBP

EBP is a term that has gained much popularity in recent years. EBP is a movement toward an increased assimilation of newly generated research evidence into direct patient care delivery and has influenced the healthcare sector for over two decades. However, it is a complex issue and has been defined and redefined many times.

Put simply, EBP is practice that is supported by a clear up-to-date rationale, taking into account the patients' preferences and using professional judgment. Sackett et al. (1996:71) defined EBP as 'the conscientious, explicit and judicious use of current best evidence in making decisions about the care of individual patients'. They assert that good doctors, and we could now replace this phrase with 'good healthcare professionals', should use both their clinical expertise or skills and the best available evidence to provide the best care for their patients. They further state that neither alone, that is, evidence or care, is enough and that best available evidence needs to be taken in context, in that it may be inappropriate for an individual patient. Equally, practice becomes outdated if there is no reference to current best evidence. Further than this, though, is the need to remember that EBP is not only an amalgamation of scientific evidence and clinical expertise, but must also reflect the patients' needs and choices. In a more recent definition, Dawes et al. (2005: 2), in the Sicily statement, offer a softer and more holistic definition of EBP:

> Evidence based practice requires that decisions about healthcare are based on the best available current valid and relevant evidence. These decisions should be made by those receiving care, informed by the tacit and explicit knowledge of those providing care, within the context of available resources.

As can be seen, the focus has changed somewhat, and in the definition Dawes et al. (2005) the emphasis for the decision-making is placed with the patient rather than the health or social care professional.

One of the criticisms of EBP, however, is that it 'ties the hands of practitioners and robs patients of their personal choices in reaching a decision about optimal care' (DaCruz 2002:674). Haynes et al. (2002) dispute this, agreeing that there are barriers to EBP, but stating that these are not two of them. They state that clinical decisions must be based on the preference of patients. In their article they posit that clinical decisions must include

1. An understanding of the patient's clinical and physical condition in order to verify what is wrong and what treatments are available
2. Research evidence that highlights the efficacy, effectiveness and efficiency of the possible treatments
3. Consideration of the patients' preferences
4. The recommendation of a treatment, which the patient accepts.

So the evidence-based prescription of anticoagulants will not be dictated merely by considering the positive effect of anticoagulation. The decision must also consider the adverse side effects and will vary from patient to patient according to their clinical and physical condition, as stated in point 1 above.

Decisions therefore vary from circumstance to circumstance and patent to patient with the same circumstance, making achieving a balance challenging. Providing information to patients in a way that enables them to make an informed decision is exacting and doctor–patient communication is key.

Activity

Where do you think the balance should lie between the health or social care provider making a decision and that decision being made by those in receipt of care? Consider the legal, ethical and professional responsibilities of the healthcare professional, for example paternalism vs. advocacy and patient autonomy, deontology vs. utilitarianism.

A further, more recent definition is given by Melnyk et al. (2008: 11) who define EBP as '. . . a problem solving approach to clinical practice that integrates a systematic search for, and critical appraisal of, the most relevant evidence to answer a burning clinical question, one's own clinical expertise, patient preferences and values.'

Activity

- What key elements do all of the definitions of EBP have in common?
- Does this fit with your understanding of EBP?

What does EBP mean to us as practitioners and consumers of healthcare?

Case study

You have planned to go on a remote trekking holiday in a country where malaria is prevalent. You attend a travel clinic to enquire about malaria prophylaxis. Unfortunately the practitioner that you see is not up to date and recommends malaria prophylaxis that is now rarely used and is largely considered to be ineffective against modern strains of malaria.

Other more effective drugs with fewer adverse side effects are now prescribed for malaria prophylaxis. However, the practitioner has been administering this older drug for years and is unaware of the newer more effective drugs. You take the older drug recommended by the practitioner.

The practitioner in the case study is not practising EBP because they are not using the best up-to-date evidence to inform their practice. As a result the practitioner is putting your health at risk.

Accountability

As a healthcare professional you are accountable. This means that you have a professional responsibility to justify and give a clear account of, and rationale for, your practice. Failure to do this may result in professional misconduct. We are accountable not only to our professional body but are also accountable to the law.

Activity

- As an accountable healthcare professional what elements of your professional code of conduct support the use of EBP?

Could the practitioner in this case study justify and give a clear account and rationale for their practice? We can see that when you are called to account for your practice you will only be able to do so if you have administered care that is based on the best available evidence. You will not be able to account for care that is based on old or weak evidence.

If there is a standard or a policy document in the practitioner's place of work that recommended the newer malaria prophylaxis, then the practitioner would find it difficult to justify administering the old medication. Even if no such documentation existed, the practitioner would still find it difficult to justify why an outdated medication was administered when a more effective medication was available.

The link between EBP, quality assurance and clinical governance

Quality is both a vision and an attribute in healthcare. We gave a number of definitions of quality in chapter 1, but it is also important to remember that quality assurance in healthcare is also high on the global agenda.

The World Organization of Family Doctors for Asia (WONCA) define quality assurance as a process of planned activities based on performance review and enhancement with the aim of continually improving standards of patient care (WONCA 2005).

Quality assurance is a means of ensuring that practitioners are engaging in best practice and that patients are receiving the best possible care. It involves looking at the delivery of healthcare in your own practice through activities such as clinical audit, review of preventative care activities, survey of patient satisfaction, and review of practice organization. It is a way of identifying areas for further education or for making useful changes in the practice.

In recent years, amidst other attempts, clinical governance has emerged to become an effective approach to pursuing quality of care. The UK National Health Service defined clinical governance as 'a framework through which organizations are accountable for continuously improving the quality of their services and safeguarding high standards of care by creating an environment in which excellence in clinical care will flourish' (Department of Health UK 2013, no page number).

As discussed in chapter 1, the key components of clinical governance are a comprehensive quality improvement programme, arrangements for continuing professional development, policies for managing risk and tackling poor performance and clear lines of accountability for the quality of care.

Activity

Consider the case study above. How could clinical governance activities ensure that the practitioner administered the correct malaria prophylaxis?

Litigation and negligence

Another reason why it is important that you can justify the care that you give is that this may protect the healthcare professional or the healthcare organization from litigation. As discussed previously, there is a developing culture of litigation and claims against healthcare organizations. Patients or clients who are unhappy about the care they receive can make a claim in negligence if they have suffered harm as a result of that care.

> ### Activity
>
> Consider the case study again. Imagine that the worse does happen and you contract malaria during your remote trek. You become very ill and are unable to work during your illness and recovery period. What laws are in place to protect you? How would the legal system support you in getting compensation?

Defining the problem: using PICO

What do you want to know? If you are looking for evidence to inform your practice (to improve it or to confirm that it is the best that it can be), then you will need to ask an answerable question.

The PICO tool (Polit and Beck 2013) is useful to ensure that your question is answerable:

P: Patient or population
I: Intervention or indicator
C: Comparison or control
O: Outcome

Thinking about falls in the elderly, you might wish to know how to reduce falls in hospitalized confused elderly:

P: How would you describe your population or patient?
     For the older confused patient on bed rest. . .
I: What Intervention or Indicator (therapy, diagnostic test or exposure) are you interested in?
     . . . is fitting bed safety rails preferable
C: What alternative or different option do you want to compare your intervention to?
     . . . to not fitting them
O: What measurable outcome(s) are you interested in?
     . . . in the interest of reducing injury.

Put together, the question is *For the older confused patient on bed rest, is fitting bed safety rails preferable to not fitting them in the interests of reducing injury?*

The above question focuses on an intervention but sometimes we are more interested in the meaning or perceptions for a particular individual group or community.

For example if we wanted to explore the attitude of carers to using safety rails for older people, then the PICO would be as follows:

P: Patient or population
I: Issue
C: Context
O: Outcome

P: How would you describe your population or patient?
    For the older confused patient on bed rest
I: What issue are you interested in?
    . . . the fitting of bed rails
C: What context?
    . . . safety
O: What outcomes?
    . . . the attitudes of carers

Put together the question is:
    For the older confused patient on bed rest what are the attitudes of carers for fitting of bed rails?

Using PICO is not an easy skill, but it will help you devise a clearly focused research question and will make your quest for relevant research much easier. Having established your question, you need to search systematically for current literature to answer it.

> **Activity**
>
> Use PICO to formulate a question related to your practice.

Finding the evidence: accessing information

The internet affords us access to huge rafts of information, but we need to learn how to access relevant academic sources. Ideally, before you access the databases available to you, it is wise to plan your search on paper.

Thinking about the older confused patient in the example above, you might wish to carry out a search on the effectiveness of drug therapy in the management of Alzheimer's disease.

> **Activity**
>
> What would be the PICO for this topic?

The question is, 'How effective is drug therapy in the management of Alzheimer's disease?'

This question has three key words/phrases:

1. Alzheimer's disease
2. Drug therapy
3. Management.

Having determined your key words, think of synonyms (words that are the same as, or similar to, your key terms). Using a dictionary or thesaurus will help you do this. Using the Boolean method of searching for literature requires the use of key words, plus the words AND, OR and NOT in combination and with a variety of other techniques, for example truncation.

Using the word OR prompts you to find key words that are similar to your first key word, for example Alzheimer's OR dementia. When AND is used, a search is narrowed, for example combining the key words Alzheimer's disease AND drug therapy will give fewer hits than merely using the phrase Alzheimer's disease. Truncation * helps expand a search. Depending on the search engine or database, the symbol may be *, ? or #. Table 6.1 illustrates a Boolean search you might use to explore the literature in a systematic way to answer your question.

Table 6.1 Example of a Boolean search

Alzheimer* disease	Drug Therap*	Manag*
Neurological Disorder*	Drug*	Treat*
Dementia	Medicat*	
Elderly Mental Health	Psychiatric Disorders – Drug Therap*	

There are many databases available, for example:

- British Nursing Index (BNI). The Royal College of Nursing provides information on how to search the BNI at http://www.rcn.org.uk/elibrary
- PubMed, which has extensive guidelines on how to search the database on its site: http://www.nlm.nih.gov/bsd/disted/pubmed.html
- The Cumulative Index to Nursing and Allied Health Literature (CINAHL) is useful for nurses and allied health professionals: http://www.cinahl.com
- The Cochrane Library provides independent high-quality evidence of healthcare decision-making. Cochrane Reviews provide systematic reviews of primary research and are internationally recognized as the highest standard in evidence-based healthcare and can be found at http://www.cochrane.org

Recording your searching strategy

Once you have undertaken a systematic electronic literature search, you should have a reasonable selection of articles, which are relevant to your research question. As mentioned before, it may be helpful to keep a record of your searching strategy and the key words that you used so that you can demonstrate a systematic approach that is the most likely to yield relevant literature for your topic. If you are searching for articles of primary research but are failing to identify these, you should document this fact. It is more accurate to write 'I did not find any literature on X' than to state categorically 'there is no literature . . .'

What counts as evidence in EBP?

Take the following example of the many things we need to consider when searching for a pair of perfect shoes. I have a formal wedding to go to next month. And I need to buy a new pair of shoes. To do this, I will need a strategy to make sure the shoes I purchase are the right ones. I will need to think about many factors:

- Are they within my budget? (Feasibility)
- Are they right for the purpose or occasion? (Appropriateness)
- Are they comfortable? (Effectiveness)
- Do I like them? (Meaningfulness)

Whether buying shoes or making a clinical decision, there are many things to consider. The same set of criteria such as feasibility, appropriateness, effectiveness and meaningfulness may apply to a clinical scenario.

Let us consider the use of Thrombo-Embolic Deterrent (TED) stockings in the post-operative prevention of deep-vein thrombosis (DVT). Research evidence suggests that TED stockings are cost effective, convenient and to have minimal side effects, making them feasible, appropriate and effective in the prevention of post-operative DVTs. However, if the patient's experience (meaningfulness) of TED stockings is that they are tight and uncomfortable to wear and they refuse to wear them, the other three factors are compromised. EBP is therefore more complex than at first sight.

Types of evidence

So what different types of evidence influence our choices? Does one type of evidence take precedence over another?

There are many different types of evidence available to underpin our clinical practice. The different types are listed in table 6.2.

Quantitative research

Quantitative research is the systematic scientific investigation of quantitative properties of phenomena and their relationships (Polit and Beck 2013). The objective of quantitative research is to develop and employ *mathematical models*, *theories* and/or *hypotheses* pertaining to natural phenomena. The

Table 6.2 Research methodologies

Quantitative research	Qualitative research
Randomized controlled trials (RCTs) Cohort and case controlled studies Cross-sectional studies/questionnaires/surveys	Grounded theory Phenomenology Ethnography Action research

Other sources
Discussion articles
Opinion
Clinical guidelines

process of measurement is central to quantitative research because it provides the fundamental connection between empirical observation and mathematical expression of quantitative relationships.

Quantitative methods (Polit and Beck 2013) include

- the generation of models, theories and hypotheses
- the development of instruments and methods for measurement
- experimental control and manipulation of variables
- collection of empirical data
- modelling and analysis of data
- evaluation of results.

The key characteristics of quantitative research are detailed in table 6.3.

Activity

Identify the key approaches of the following quantitative research methods. In addition, for each method think of a possible study that could be carried out in your area of practice.

- Randomized control trial
- Quasi experiment
- Cohort study
- Survey/questionnaire

Qualitative research

The principle of all qualitative approaches is to explore the meaning of and develop in-depth understanding of the research topic as experienced by the

Table 6.3 Philosophical underpinnings of positivist research

Paradigms	Ontology	Epistemology
Positivism	Objective	Reductionist
Post-positivism	Realist	Logico-reductionist
		Deterministic
		Causal-mechanistic
		frameworks
		Theory testing
		Political

Research methods	Data collection	Data analysis
Experiments	Instruments as data	Basic unit of
Surveys	collection tools	analysis is
Structure or non-participant		numbers
observation		Statistical analysis
Control of variables		

Rigour
Reliability
Internal validity
External validity/generalizability
Objectivity

(Pollt and Beck 2013)

participants of the research. Qualitative research seeks to understand human behaviour and the social processes in which we engage. Depth rather than breadth is the focus of qualitative research.

The key characteristics of qualitative research are detailed in table 6.4.

Activity

Identify the key approaches of the following qualitative research method. In addition, for each method think of a possible study that could be carried out in your area of practice.

- Grounded theory
- Ethnography
- Phenomenology
- Action Research

Many believe that EBP is synonymous to using research (Saad 2008, French 2002). While critical appraisal and the use of research are integral to the

Table 6.4 Philosophical underpinnings of naturalistic research

Paradigms	Ontology	Epistemology
Naturalism	Subjective	Holistic
Critical theory	Relativist	Dialectic
		Inductive
		Speculative
		Meaning
		Interpretative
		Constructivist
		Theory generating
Research methods	**Data collection**	**Data analysis**
Interviews	Listening	Basic unit of analysis is words
Focus groups	Talking	Interpretation
Observations	Observing	Thematic analysis
Rigour		
Authenticity		
Transferability		
Auditability		
Trustworthiness		

process of EBP, the process itself is much greater and more patient-centred than research use alone.

Fineout-Overholt et al. (2010) describe four sources of evidence: research, clinical experience, patient experience and information from the local context. Fineout-Overholt et al. (2010) argue that although research evidence has been traditionally viewed as the gold standard, it is not certain, acontextual and static but is dynamic and eclectic and therefore on its own is not enough to inform clinical decisions effectively. Knowledge accrued from professional practice, patient/client experience and the local context is also valued in EBP. It is evident that sometimes the different sources of evidence make uncomfortable bedfellows; however, if person/patient centred care is to be a reality, an accord between different sources of evidence needs to be found.

Hierarchy of evidence

Levels of evidence or a hierarchy (table 6.5) of evidence is a term used to reflect the methodological rigour of studies. A study assigned as level 1 evidence is considered the most rigorous and least susceptible to bias, while a study deemed to be level 8 evidence is considered the least rigorous and is more susceptible to bias.

Table 6.5 Hierarchy of evidence

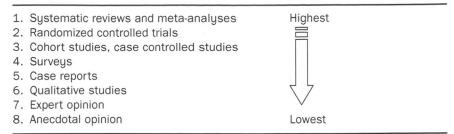

1. Systematic reviews and meta-analyses	Highest
2. Randomized controlled trials	
3. Cohort studies, case controlled studies	
4. Surveys	
5. Case reports	
6. Qualitative studies	
7. Expert opinion	
8. Anecdotal opinion	Lowest

(Adapted from Sackett et al. 1999)

Levels of evidence (Sackett et al. 1996)

There is general agreement that a hierarchy of evidence exists and that some forms of research evidence are stronger than others in addressing different types of questions. However, the hierarchy depends on the question you need to have answered.

For example if you wanted to find out whether glove use was more effective than hand washing in the prevention of the spread of hospital acquired infections, you would find stronger evidence from a randomized controlled trial that looked at a comparison between the two approaches than in a study that asked the opinion of patients or clients as to which method they thought was more effective in preventing the spread of infection. The stronger evidence provided by the RCT in this instance indicates that the RCT should be placed higher up in a hierarchy than a study exploring patients' perception of hand hygiene when addressing this particular question.

In the hierarchy of evidence, the higher up a methodology is ranked, the more robust and close to objective truth it is assumed to be. One of the most well known hierarchies of evidence that is concerned with ranking the strength of evidence relating to the effectiveness of a treatment or intervention is that developed by Sackett et al. (1996) as shown above.

However, it is also important to bear in mind that it is not always possible or desirable to undertake a RCT, even if this type of evidence is considered to be required. For example, for researchers looking at infant nutrition, it would not be acceptable or ethical to ask one group of mothers to abstain from breastfeeding their babies as a control group for another group of mothers who were asked to breastfeed.

In many areas of health and social care, the traditional hierarchy is not appropriate for exploring complex questions. You are not only interested in finding out whether something is effective; there are many other questions you need to address.

Not all scholars agree with the approach of assigning a hierarchy to evidence. Some authors suggest that this approach is dangerous and may even subjugate nursing knowledge and practices.

Critically appraising the evidence

Once you have decided what you want to know and you have searched for evidence using an appropriate search strategy, you then need to weigh up how good the evidence is and what it means.

Critical appraisal has been described as the process of systematically examining research evidence to assess its validity, results and relevance before using it to inform a decision (Hill and Spittlehouse 2003). In order to do this it is necessary to have a basic understanding of the different methodological approaches that may be taken within a research study, as this will help you to choose the correct critical appraisal tools.

The skills of critical appraisal are relatively easy to acquire and there are many tools to help you, but it is important to consider the most appropriate tools to use to appraise an individual piece of research critically. One study identified 121 published critical appraisal tools located on the internet and electronic databases (Katrak et al. 2004). This raises the issue of which tool to use for a particular paper. Many critical appraisal tools have been developed for the review of specific types of research, and as such are design specific, for example for the review of randomized controlled trials only. Other critical appraisal tools are generic and suitable for all types of research. At first glance, the reviewer might be tempted to use a critical appraisal tool that is generic to all types of research, especially if the literature searching strategy has identified many different approaches to research. However, the reviewer does need to assess the quality and appropriate application of the critical appraisal tool. Once you become engaged in the process, you will probably come to the conclusion that most research contains flaws but you will also be able to decide whether or not a piece of research has value in supporting your decision-making.

Issues and challenges

Since the 1990s, Evidence Based Practice has moved rapidly from a niche interest to a mainstream initiative, but does the reality match the theory and what are the issues that could prevent its full implementation? If we can understand these, then we may be able to find ways of overcoming them.

As discussed earlier in this chapter, there are many drivers for Evidence Based Practice, among these are the clinical governance and quality agenda as well as the need to follow the Code of Professional Conduct and Code of Ethics for nurses. The Healthcare Professions Council (HCPC) lays out the Code of Conduct for paramedics; the Chartered Society of Physiotherapists (CSP) lays out the Code of Conduct for physiotherapists; the College of Occupational Therapists provides the Code of Ethics for occupational therapists and the College of Operating Department Practitioners provides the code for operating department practitioners. These drivers often require the healthcare professional to challenge traditional practice as well as outdated policies and guidelines.

Activity

You have had an outbreak of Norovirus in your clinical area and are aware that the most effective way of preventing further spread of infection is through hand washing. Your nursing colleagues wash their hands between patients; however, you notice that the doctors are not attending to this simple measure. How will you address this in the interests of effective patient care?

Legal implications of Evidence Based Practice

Pearson et al. (2007) argued that as we have declared that our past practice was not based on evidence and now the EBP movement has become unstoppable, the law is taking an increasing interest in seeing that the best care is provided for patients. This increasingly litigious approach, having started in the USA, has now started to spread across the globe. Pearson et al. (2007) went on to suggest that clinical negligence is now being assessed in the courts in many countries (South Africa, Canada and America), with experts assessing and interpreting research evidence rather than the traditional expert witness. Interestingly the testimonies of expert witnesses are increasingly being challenged in the UK.

Activity

- Does practice that is not deemed to be best practice have to be regarded as negligent practice?
- What are your views?

Feasibility, appropriateness and meaningfulness

Feasibility, appropriateness and meaningfulness are important and have been outlined by Pearson et al. (2007) reminding us that a further aspect of weighing up the value of a piece of research is to start to consider the patient or population we are most interested in.

Patient values, preferences, cultural and religious beliefs will impact on their choice of an intervention we might offer them in our roles as healthcare practitioners.

Evidence and patient preference

As has been discussed earlier in this chapter, it is very important to consider the importance of patient preference in EBP. For example, a certain Calcium Alginate dressing may have stronger evidence for its use than another. However, an individual patient may prefer the alternative dressing because it results in less exudate and therefore means that the dressing is more manageable in everyday life. No matter how strong the evidence is, that patient is likely to take the dressing off when they get home and apply their own remedy. This will result in increased cost to whoever is paying for the wasted dressing and will also mean that you are spending time on carrying out needless dressings. Whatever the evidence suggests, consideration of the patients' preferences and the recommendation of a treatment, which is acceptable to the patient, are central to EBP.

Values Based Practice

No discussion on EBP is complete without a discussion on Values Based Practice (VBP), which may be defined as the sister of EBP and 'putting the values of individual service users and carers at the centre of everything we do. It also means understanding and using our own values and beliefs in a positive way and respecting the values of the other people we work with' (Woodbridge and Fulford 2003:32).

Fulford (2011) discusses the new partnership between EBP and VBP, illuminating the synergy between VBP and EBP in delivering care by incorporating a patient's values. Taking a step further than EBP, Fulford (2011) states that by incorporating a patient's unique values, such as preferences, anxieties, needs and wishes into a decision based on clinical evidence leads to patient centred medicine.

Currently VBP is predominantly embodied within the field of mental health and CCAWI (the Centre for Clinical and Academic Workforce Innovation) at the University of Lincoln has been supporting the national roll out of the ten Essential Shared Capabilities (ESC) programme. This was a Department of Health funded initiative to examine the application of VBP into partnerships with service users, carers and others working in mental health (CCAWI 2005).

Evolving policy and legislation to improve patient centred care in mental health and the increasing imperative to include values, rights and personal outcomes in care resulted in the following Essential Capabilities:

1. Working in partnership
2. Respecting diversity
3. Practising ethically
4. Challenging inequality
5. Promoting recovery, well-being and self-management
6. Identifying people's needs and strengths

7. Providing person-centred care
8. Making a difference
9. Promoting safety and risk enablement
10. Personal development and learning.

Further detail regarding the ten ESCs is given in the Department of Health (2004) framework for the mental health workforce. Appendix A of this document shows the link between ESCs, the Capable Practitioner Framework (CPF), the National Occupational Standards (NOS) and the Knowledge and Skills Framework (KSF). It is important to remember that the four frameworks were developed separately; they do not cover the same issues and the ESC, the CPF and the NOS have been developed for mental health services whilst the KSF has a NHS focus. Figure 6.1 illustrates how values, rights and personal outcomes are incorporated in the improvement of patient centred care.

Fulford (2011) adds to this diagram by stating that all clinical decisions stand on two feet: left foot, values, and right foot, evidence.

The NIMHE (National Institute for Mental Health England) lists the following framework of principles of VBP:

1. *Recognition* of the role of values alongside evidence in all areas of mental health delivery and practice
2. *Raising awareness* that values are context based, and the impact they have on practice in mental health
3. *Respect* of the diversity of values, working to ensure that the principle of service user centrality is the unifying focus for practice. By so doing the values of each service user/client and their communities must be the key determinant of all actions taken by professionals.

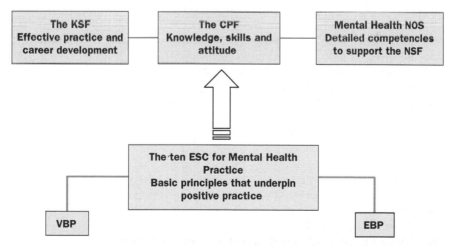

Figure 6.1 Improving patient centred care. (Woodbridge and Fulford 2003)

Respect for diversity is

- user-centred – the values of individual users are central
- recovery oriented – cultural and racial difference impact on the routes to recovery
- multidisciplinary – respect is reciprocal at an individual level, at a disciplinary level (nursing, medicine, social work) and at an organizational level (health, social care, community groups, etc.)
- dynamic – respect is responsive to change
- reflective – respect combines self-monitoring and self management
- balanced – positive and negative values are recognized
- relational – positive working relationships supported by good communication at the heart of practice.

Warwick Medical School has led on the development of VBP in mental health and primary care and is extending the approach to other areas of healthcare.

Activity

- Have you made a clinical decision recently?
- Regardless of whether you work in a mental health facility or not, was your decision based on the ten ESCs and the NIMHE's three guiding principles?
- If no, how might you incorporate these into future clinical decision-making?

In summary, Burns and Grove (2011:4) describe nursing research (to search again or to examine carefully) as a systematic and scientific inquiry that '. . . validates and refines existing knowledge and develops new knowledge that directly and indirectly influences nursing practice. Nursing research is the key to building an Evidence Based Practice for nurses.'

The ultimate goal therefore is the 'development of an empirical body of knowledge for a discipline or profession, such as nursing' (Burns and Grove 2011:4). In order for healthcare professionals to promote positive outcomes for patients and their families, they need to be able to read and understand research reports to implement Evidence Based Practice. Often this evidence will be used to formulate protocols and guidelines.

The goal of EBP is to promote quality and cost-effective outcomes for patients, their families and healthcare providers. As stated above, EBP is the integration of the best research evidence, clinical expertise and patient needs and values. The best research evidence is the empirical evidence that is generated from the synthesis of research findings to understand a problem in practice. Healthcare professionals require a solid research base in order to implement interventions to treat conditions and promote positive outcomes for both the patient and their family. In so doing, they will also ascertain that their patients receive quality care (Burns and Grove 2011).

EBP and care pathways

Integrated care pathways were briefly mentioned in table 1.2 in chapter 1 when the attributes of clinical governance were first discussed. EBP is central to the formulation of care pathways and care bundles.

Terminology varies and integrated care pathways (ICP), anticipated recovery pathways (ARP), multidisciplinary pathways of care (MPC), collaborative care programmes (CCP) are terms synonymous with each other. Swage (2004:134) defines a care pathway as follows:

An integrated care pathway determines locally agreed, multidisciplinary practice based on guidelines and evidence where available, for a specific patient/client group. It forms all or part of the clinical record, documents the care given and facilitates the evaluation of outcomes for continuous quality improvements.

Care pathways can provide patients with clear expectations of their care and are a means of measuring their progress; therefore they can be seen to maximize the quality provided at each step of the patient's journey.

They also promote teamwork by an increased understanding of the differing roles of the multidisciplinary team. Additionally they facilitate the use of guidelines (Evans-Lacko et al. 2010). For a specific patient group, a care pathway considers and maps all anticipated elements of care and all treatment provided by a multidisciplinary team of clinicians. Deviation from the pathway is noted in the patient's case notes as a variance, and variance analysis provides information on current practice. Furthermore variance analysis encourages a multidisciplinary audit, as the team are able to analyse what care was actually given compared to the care that was laid down by the care pathway. The benefits of care pathways are numerous. However, teams also need to consider the limitations, some of which are highlighted in table 6.6.

A well-written pathway can lead to consistent care of the highest quality, thus supporting the notion of clinical governance. In order to be consistent there are a number of steps that need to be included when designing a pathway (Moullin 2002, Sale 2005, Swage 2004):

1. Identify patient group.
2. Set start/finish point (e.g. admission and discharge; follow up to outpatients).
3. Agree outcomes and personnel responsible.
4. Agree timescales.
5. Ensure that dates are recorded.

Table 6.6 Critique of care pathways

Benefits of pathways	Limitations of pathways
• Integrating evidence based clinical guidelines into practice • Monitoring standards • Measuring quality • Some evidence that ICPs increase patient satisfaction • Involving all members of the multidisciplinary team • Reducing duplication • Improving consistency • Managing risk • Ensuring that treatment is evidence based • Can be used as part of audit • Considered an audit-friendly tool • Can be used to identify where there are delays in the service • Standardized and therefore can reduce variations in service provided • Some evidence on the benefits of ICPs (RCTs) • Reduce hospital complications • Reduce hospital length of stay • Improve outcomes • Reduce costs • Avoid replication of care.	• Lack of engagement of the organization, management and clinical staff • It would appear that the greatest barrier is presented by clinical staff (Evans-Lacko 2010), who may be reluctant to change • Take time to design • Could be considered inflexible • Could be considered to prevent clinical decision-making • If electronic – computer problems • Difficult to design for an individual with multiple pathologies • Require leadership and good communication to implement successfully • Lack of evidence-based guidelines.

(Pickering and Thompson 2003, Swage 2004, Sale 2005, Allen et al. 2009, Rotter et al. 2008)

6. Track variances and analyse data.
7. Feedback and review.
8. Update pathway if necessary.

Resources

The Royal College of Nursing: http://www.rcn.org.uk/development/practice/perioperative_fasting/good_practice/service_improvement_tools/care_pathways) provides more information on integrated pathways, in particular a workbook for those wishing to develop integrated care pathways.

The College of Occupational Therapy: http://www.cot.co.uk
If you type 'pathways' into the search box, you will find a number of pathways.
The Chartered Society of Physiotherapy: http://csp.org.uk/tagged/integrated-care-pathways
Here you will find a link to a care pathway for falls and osteoporosis.
Lincolnshire Care Pathway Partnership: http://mrsaactionuk.net/Lincs%20Care%20Pathway%20Project.pdf
Here you will find an integrated pathway for MRSA.

EBP and care bundles

It is essential for those working in critical care to ensure that their practices are *evidence based* (Lawrence and Fulbrook 2011), with the purpose of EBP being that existing evidence is applied to practice.

There are many forms of evidence and equally there are many ways in which evidence can be applied to practice; for example the development of evidence-based protocols or care pathways, as discussed above. Building on this, Fulbrook and Mooney (2003:250) first described care bundles in the critical care nursing literature, describing a care bundle as 'The idea is that several practices, when used in combination, or as a cluster, *all of the time*, have a greater effect on the positive outcome of patients.'

Care bundles are a collection of interventions (usually three to five) that may be applied to the management of a particular condition. *Based on evidence*, the elements in a bundle are best practices brought together into a single quality measure (Aboelela et al. 2007). We discussed ventilator-acquired pneumonia (VAP) in chapter 2, and Lawrence and Fulbrook (2011) suggest that a reduction in VAP is associated with VCB (ventilator care bundle) use and represents best practice for all eligible adult ventilated patients in intensive care.

Resource

High impact intervention. Care bundle to reduce ventilation-association: http://tinyurl.com/m2aw6qz

Berenholtz et al. (2002) hypothesized the notion of bundling a number of interventions, with each intervention being based on strong evidence. In their study, they reviewed the literature between 1964 and 2000 and identified six outcome measures and six process measures that provided a measure of quality of intensive care. Four of the measures were grouped together by the

Joint Commission on Accrediting of Healthcare Organisations (JCAHO) to form the VAP VCB:

1. Elevation of the head of the bed
2. Daily interruption of sedation to assess readiness to wean
3. Gastric ulcer prevention
4. Deep vein thrombosis prophylaxis (DVTP).

The four elements of the Berenholtz's VCB were based on highest-level evidence, that is, systematic reviews of randomized control trials (RCTs) and single RCTs.

The VCB was tested in a 14-bed ICU for one year (Berenholtz et al. 2004) and showed a decreased mortality if all four elements were applied. The Institute of Health Improvement conducted a multi-centre study in ICUs in the USA and Canada from 2002 to 2004, investigating the relationship between compliance with the VCB and its effect on clinical outcomes (O'Keefe-McCarthy et al. 2008). The study was significant because it demonstrated that VCB reduced ventilator days and ICU length of stay as well as dramatically reducing VAP rates.

Further research (DuBose et al. 2008, Khorfan 2008) suggest the addition of oral care to the original four elements.

Lawrence and Fulbrook (2011) were unable to prove the link between VCB and VAP incidence and length of ventilation and ICU length of stay, but a strong relationship is suggested.

Further resources:

Pressure ulcer prevention and management care bundle:
    www.cmccn.nhs.uk/about/policies/document/North_West_Critical_
    Care_Networks_SKIN_Bundle
FallSafe care bundle:
    www.rcplondon.ac.uk/sites/default. . ./fallsafe-care-bundles.pdf

---

Activity

- Have you used either an integrated care pathway or a care bundle?
- How helpful were they?

Key point summary

EBP and VBP are fundamental to improving clinical practice. A necessary part of EBP is to define a problem, preferably using PICO and access information (or evidence) in order to address the problem.

- Integrated care pathways, whilst not essential, enable multidisciplinary teams to work together to provide excellent patient care at each stage of the patient's journey. ICPs highlight variance that should be identified through audit. They also provide information to patients/service users on how their treatment will be managed.
- Care bundles are a collection of interventions that can be applied to the management of a particular condition.

Implications for practice

- All healthcare professionals must be accountable for their practice, and best practice includes appreciating the evidence.
- Staff need to be aware of the limitations of integrated care pathways and care bundles.

End-of-chapter questions

1. Why are EBP and VBP essential to clinical practice?
2. When examining your practice, what is the tool to help you ask an answerable question to ensure your practice is evidence based?
3. What do the letters stand for?
4. What is the difference between an integrated care pathway and a care bundle?

See the Appendix on page 193 for suggested answers to these questions.

References

Aboelela SW, Stone PW and Larson L (2007) Effectiveness of bundled behavioural interventions to control healthcare-associated infections: A systematic review of the literature. *Journal of Hospital Infection*, 66, 101–108

Allen D, Gillen E and Rixon L (2009) Systematic review of the effectiveness of integrated care pathways: What works, for whom, in what circumstances? *International Journal of Evidence-based Healthcare*, 7 (2), 61–74

Berenholtz S, Dorman T, Ngo K, Provonest P (2002) Qualitative review of intensive care quality indicators. *Journal of Critical Care*, 17, 1–12

Berenholtz SM, Milanovich S, Faircloth A, Prow DI, Earsing K, Lipsett P, Dorman T and Pronovost PJ (2004) Improving care for the ventilated patient. *Joint Commission Journal on Quality and Safety*, 30, 195–204

Burns N and Grove SK (2011) *Understanding nursing research: Building an evidence based practice* (5th ed.). Maryland Heights: Saunders

CCAWI (2005) The Centre for Clinical and Academic Workforce Innovation www.lincoln.ac.uk/ xx_Archive/ccawi/ (accessed 16.12.2013)

Da Cruz D (2002) You have a choice dear patient. *British Medical Journal*, 324, 674

Dawes M, Summerskill W, Glasziou P, Cartabellotta A, Martin J, Hopyian K, Porzsolt F, Burks A, Osbourne J (2005) Sicily statement on Evidence Based Practice. *BMC Medical Education*, 5 (1), 1–7

Department of Health (2004) The ten essential shared capabilities: A framework for the whole of the mental health workforce. London: Department of Health

Department of Health (2013) Making the NHS more efficient and less bureaucratic. Available at https://www.gov.uk/government/policies/making-the-NHS-more-efficient-and-less-bureaucratic (accessed 12.12.2013)

DuBose JJ, Inaba K, Shiflett A, Trankiem C, Teixeira PGR, Salim A, Rhee P, Demitriades D, Belzberg H (2008) Measurable outcomes of quality improvement in the trauma intensive care unit: The impact of a daily quality rounding checklist. *Journal of Trauma, Injury, Infection and Critical Care*, 64, 22–29

Evans-Lacko S, Jarrett M, McCrone P and Thornicroft G (2010) Facilitators and barriers to implementing clinical care pathways. *BMC Health Services Research*, 182 doi: 10.1186/1472-6963-10-182

Fineout-Overholt E, Melnyck BM, Stillwell SB (2010) Evidence-based practice, step by step: Critical appraisal of the evidence, part 1. *American Journal of Nursing*, 110 (7), 47–52

Fulbrook P and Mooney S (2003) Care bundles in critical care: A practical approach to Evidence Based Practice. *Nursing in Critical Care*, 8, 249–255

Fulford K W M (2011) The value of evidence and evidence of values: Bringing together value based and Evidence Based Practice in policy and service development in mental health. *Journal of Evaluation Clinical Practice*, 17 (5), 976–987

Haynes RB, Devereaux PJ and Guyatt GH (2002) Physicians' and patients' choices in Evidence Based Practice. *British Medical Journal*, 324, 1350

Hill A and Spittlehouse C (2003) Evidence based medicine – what is critical appraisal? Newmarket: Hayward Medical Communications

Katrak P, Bialocerkowski AE, Massy-Westropp N, Kumar VSSS and Grimmer KA (2004) A systematic review of the content of critical appraisal tools. *BMC Medical Research Methodology*, 4 (22), 17–29

Khorfan F (2008) Daily goals checklist – a goal directed method to eliminate nosocomial infection in the intensive care unit. *Journal for Healthcare Quality*, 30, 13–17

Lawrence P and Fulbrook P (2011) The ventilator care bundle and its impact on ventilator-associated pneumonia: A review of the evidence. *Nursing in Critical Care*, 15 (5), 222–234

Melnyk BM, Fineout-Overholt E, Feinstein NF, Sadler LS, Green-Hernandez C (2008) Nurse practitioner educators' perceived knowledge, beliefs, and teaching strategies regarding Evidence Based Practice: Implications for accelerating the integration of Evidence Based Practice into graduate programs. *Journal of Professional Nursing*, 24 (1), 7–13

Moullin M (2003) *Delivering excellence in health and social care*. Maidenhead: Open University Press

O'Keefe-McCarthy S, Santiago C, Lau G (2008) Ventilator-associated pneumonia bundled strategies: An Evidence Based Practice. *Worldviews on Evidence-Based Nursing*, 5 (4), 193–204

Pearson A, Field J and Jordan Z (2007) *Evidence-based clinical practice in nursing and healthcare: Assimilating research, experience and expertise*. Oxford: Blackwell

Pickering S and Thompson J (2003) *Clinical governance and best value*. London: Churchill Livingstone

Polit DF and Beck CT (2013) *Essentials of nursing research: Appraising evide. nursing practice.* Philadelphia: Lippincott, Williams and Wilkins

Rotter T, Kugler J, Koch R, Gothe H, Twork S, Van Oostrum J and Steyerberg E (2008) A systematic review and meta-analysis of the effects of clinical pathways on length of stay, hospital costs and patient outcomes. *BMC Health Service Research*, 8, 265–280

Sackett DL, Rosenberg WM, Muir Gray JA and Richardson WS (1996) Evidence based medicine: What it is and what it isn't. *British Medical Journal*, 312, 71–72

Sale D (2005) *Understanding clinical governance and quality assurance: Making it happen.* Basingstoke: Palgrave Macmillan

Swage T (2004) *Clinical governance in health care practice.* Oxford: Butterworth Heinemann

WONCA (2005) *Quality assurance.* Available at http://www.pdqa.gov.hk/english/qa/qa.php (accessed 03.12.2013)

Woodbridge K and Fulford KWM (2003) Good practice? Values based practice in mental health. *Mental Health Practice*, 7 (2), 30–33

7

Implementing clinical governance through risk and complaints management

Gail E Lansdown

Chapter contents

- Learning objectives
- Introduction
- Quality control (QC), quality assurance (QA), total quality management (TQM) and continuous quality improvement (CQI)
- Clinical risk and risk management
- The link between risk management and quality assurance
- Complaints management
- Empowering patients/service users and staff to enable them to shape governance strategies collaboratively (shared governance)
- Key point summary
- Implications for practice
- End-of-chapter questions
- References

Let's begin by thinking back to Som's definition (2004:89) of quality control:

> A governance system for healthcare organizations that promotes an integrated approach towards management of inputs, structures and processes to improve the outcome of the healthcare service delivery where health staff work in an environment of greater accountability for clinical quality.

Learning objectives

This chapter will enable the reader to have a better understanding of

- quality control (QC), quality assurance (QA) and total quality management (TQM)/continuous quality improvement (CQI)
- clinical risk
- risk management cycle: risk identification, analysis, control and evaluation
- complaints management, local resolution, independent review
- learning from complaints
- empowering patients/service users and staff to enable them to shape governance strategies collaboratively (shared governance).

Introduction

Chapter 5 introduced the concept of implementing clinical governance strategies through education and training. This chapter will focus on quality control, the use of risk management and complaints management to implement clinical governance.

Quality control (QC), quality assurance (QA), total quality management (TQM) and continuous quality improvement (CQI)

Quality control is key in clinical governance, and it is widely believed that there are four approaches to quality:

1. Quality control (QC)
2. Total quality management (TQM)
3. Continuous quality improvement (CQI)
4. Quality assurance (QA).

We now look at each approach in turn.

Quality control (QC)

The fundamentals of quality control have been in evidence, either directly or indirectly, for centuries. The Greeks and Egyptians set standards in their construction, arts and crafts. In the Middle Ages and up to the nineteenth century, goods were manufactured in the main by individuals or small groups and so the notion of *operator quality control* was labelled by Feigenbaum (1983).

The term *foreman quality control* was conceived by Feigenbaum (1983) to denote the quality control of items produced in the early twentieth century (and continuing until approximately 1920) during the Industrial Revolution. This term was coined to denote the fact that a supervisor or foreman oversaw the quality of goods.

From 1920 to the 1940s, production and processes became more complex, standards were set and foreman quality control gave way to *inspector quality control* (Feigenbaum 1983). In the 1930s, sampling became the norm rather than a 100% scrutiny of products, particularly as this was not feasible during the period of the Second World War. Feigenbaum (1983) terms this period (1930s to 1960s) *statistical quality control*. Quality control gained attention in England in the 1930s and the British Standards Institution Standard 600 dealt with applications of statistical methods of quality control (Mitra 2012). The American Society for Quality Control was formed in 1946, and Japan seized the notion of statistical quality control with enthusiasm in 1950.

Named again by Feigenbaum (1983) the next phase, *total quality control* (or Total Quality Management), came into being in the 1960s. At this time, quality control moved away from the inspection department and became the remit of manufacturing departments as manufacturers realized that each department had a role to play in the production of a quality article. At the same time, quality circles gained popularity in Japan (discussed in chapter 3).

The 1970s saw the advent of the *total quality control organizationwide phase*, involving the participation of all members of the company (Feigenbaum 1983). The *total quality system* was born in the 1980s (Feigenbaum 1983).

The 1970s saw the growing use of the cause-and-effect diagram, also known as the Ishikawa diagram (chapter 3). First introduced in 1946, it gained increasing popularity at this time as a tool able to identify possible reasons as to why a process might become uncontrolled and the possible impacts of this. During the 1970s, Taguchi from Japan introduced the concept of quality improvement through statistically designed experiments (Mitra 2012).

As computer use increased ubiquitously in the 1980s, the market was flooded with quality control software. As the emphasis on customer satisfaction and quality improvement became greater globally, so increased the need for a system to support the quality agenda, and the International Organization for Standardization (ISO) was formed.

The evolution of the information technology era could possibly be described as the greatest revolution since the Industrial Revolution (Mitra 2012). The internet has raised expectations in that service providers will be expected to transact an error-free transaction from production or provision of a service to delivery. According to Mitra (2012:7), '. . . the current century will continue to experience a thrust in growth of quality assurance and improvement methods that can, using technology, assimilate data and analyse them in real time and with no tolerance for errors.'

Healthcare organizations

Quality control in healthcare organizations refers to activities that evaluate, monitor or regulate services provided to consumers in which processes are observed, characteristics are identified and variables are tracked through statistical methods (Mitra 2012).

The following steps should be taken to monitor and evaluate performance in healthcare services:

1. Control criteria are established.
2. Information relevant to the criteria are identified.
3. Information collection is agreed.
4. Information is collected and analysed.
5. Collected information is compared with control criteria.
6. Judgement made about quality.
7. Corrective action taken if necessary.
8. Re-evaluate.

Total quality management (TQM) and continuous quality improvement (CQI)

McLaughlin and Kaluzny (2006) posit that TQM and CQI are one and the same thing and both are terms depicting the planning and execution of a flow of improvement to provide quality care that meets or exceeds expectation.

McLaughlin and Kaluzny (2006) suggest that TQM/CQI have similar char-acteristics:

1. A link to the organization's strategic plan
2. A quality council of staff from the highest level
3. Training programmes
4. Mechanisms for choosing areas for improvement
5. The formation of improvement teams
6. Policies that support and motivate staff to take part in improvement pro-cesses.

Improvements can take place at three levels:

1. *Localized improvements* – when an ad hoc team meets to focus on a particular problem or opportunity
2. *Organizational learning* – the development of policies and procedures, for example protocols or clinical pathways (chapter 6)
3. *Process re-engineering* – major investment supports the radical amendment to organizational process.

They suggest that TQM refers to industry-based programmes, whereas CQI refers to clinical settings.

According to McLaughlin and Kaluzny (2006), CQI comes in a variety of forms but does have a number of essential characteristics:

1. Understanding and responding to the organization's external environment
2. Empowering clinicians and managers to make improvements
3. Acknowledging that customers (patients and providers) are the primary determinants of quality
4. Moving away from departmental and professional silos to a multidisciplinary ethos
5. Instituting a planned and agreed philosophy of change and adaptation
6. Ensuring best practice through organizational learning
7. Supporting a rational, data-based approach to analysis and change.

Therefore CQI is both a management philosophy and a management method.

Quality assurance (QA)

As described above, quality is no longer the responsibility of one person (operator quality control). In the current age, everyone under the total quality system, or TQM/CQI, is now responsible for quality, whether directly or indirectly. Unfortunately, as has been shown in recent reports (e.g. the Francis Report), something that should be everyone's responsibility becomes no one's responsibility, thus creating an inefficient and ineffective system where quality appears to be given merely lip service. Quality Assurance is a system whereby all procedures that have been designed and planned are followed (Mitra 2012). The quality assurance function should continually survey the quality philosophy of the organization, with the quality assurance team auditing all areas to discover and correct errors.

Healthcare

Quality assurance in healthcare should objectively and systematically monitor and evaluate the quality of patient care, improve patient care where possible and resolve problems as required. The QA process requires a definition of quality, a measurement of quality and an improvement of quality.

Activity

- How does your workplace address quality issues?
- Which of the processes above are followed (McLaughlin and Kaluzny 2006)?
- How well are they followed?

Key points

- Quality control is key in clinical governance.
- It is widely believed there are four approaches to quality: (1) QC, (2) TQM, (3) QA, (4) CQI.
- McLaughlin and Kaluzny (2006) suggest that TQM and CQI have similar characteristics.

Clinical risk and risk management

Due to its unpredictability, healthcare is risky (e.g. human error, adverse events and systems failures), and to ameliorate this, risk management is key. It has been defined as the systematic identification, assessment and evaluation of risk (Cottee and Harding 2008). Fenn and Egan (2012:25) argue that not only can risk management be used as an incident-reporting tool, but it can also be used 'to reduce the risk that clinical or resourcing errors can cause to patients and staff'. Several key reports (Department of Health 2000, 2004) highlighting the need to learn from clinical error and improvement to quality of care respectively have been instrumental in emphasizing the importance and development of risk management.

Risk management is integral to clinical governance, described by Chandraharan and Arulkumaran (2007:223) as

a framework through which NHS organizations are accountable for continuously improving the quality of their services and safeguarding high standards of care by creating an environment in which excellence in clinical care will flourish.

Furthermore, many elements of risk management are integral to clinical governance, for example:

- risk reporting, including response to complaints
- audit
- guidelines
- risk assessment
- training.

Although not fully instigated until 2000, a risk management programme was implemented in 1995 by the NHS Litigation Authority (NHSLA) (Fenn and Egan 2012) and Trusts are subject to audit by NHSLA in order to maintain their membership of the Clinical Negligence Scheme for Trusts (CNST). Simplistically, risk management encompasses the identification, assessment and reduction of risks to patients, visitors, staff and organizational assets. Risk management can also be seen as a programme to reduce preventable accidents and injuries, thereby reducing the financial loss to the organization should an accident or injury occur (Smith and Wheeler 1992). Bluntly, risk management is the protection of assets, and those in charge of risk management manage this by

1. Risk identification
2. Risk analysis
3. Risk control or treatment
4. Risk financing.

Risk identification

Important to remember that this is not a single assessment of risk but an ongoing process, risk identification involves the identification of past and current patient care incidents and other events that may present a potential loss to the organization (Kavaler and Spiegel 2003). The identification of possible liability risks such as unexpected treatment outcomes, complaints and adverse events must be an ongoing process.

Risk analysis

This involves the evaluation of past and current episodes in order to assess the probable severity to the individual and the organization, the number of people possibly harmed and the likelihood or frequency of the occurrence.

Risk control or treatment

This is the organization's response to significant risk areas and is the most common function of risk management programmes. Kavaler and Spiegel (2003) list a combination of techniques for controlling risk:

1. *Risk acceptance* – the organization takes a measured decision not to purchase insurance against a particular adverse event.
2. *Exposure avoidance* – removing the service, personnel or equipment that may cause the loss.
3. *Loss prevention* – improve education for staff; improve communication with patients when a mishap occurs in the hope that this will produce a satisfied patient who will not sue the organization.
4. *Loss reduction* – education, revision of policies and procedures.
5. *Exposure segregation* – separate out the 'offending' service, for example in the case of medication errors, all drugs can be dispensed from a central location.
6. *Contractual transfer* – contract the service out to another provider.

Activity

Thinking about the drug trial in 2006 where TGN1412 was used in a clinical trial. This was a clinical trial in which six young men went into organ failure hours after taking TGN1412.

* How might the six points above impact on further drug trials?

Whilst drug trials such as TGN1412 are essential in the acceptance of new treatments, organizations managing these trials have to control the risk. They have a responsibility to ensure that risk is mitigaged through treatment of potential side effects and have to ensure that finances are available for compensation.

Risk financing

Risk financing requires an understanding and evaluation of the finances involved, for example insurance, liability payouts.

In the USA, the American Society of Healthcare Risk Management (ASHRM) offers a risk management programme (Kavaler and Spiegel 2003) in which

1. There will be a designated risk manager who will receive at least eight hours of risk management training annually
2. Risk managers will have access to all data, whether medical or management
3. A written policy statement regarding risk management will be agreed by the governing body, the medical staff and administration of the organization
4. There will be a system to identify, review and analyse all adverse outcomes, unanticipated or otherwise
5. Risk management data will be centralized
6. A report from the risk manager will be presented annually to the governing body of the organization
7. Risk managers will ensure that all medical staff and new employees attend educational programmes on minimizing clinical risk and high-risk clinical areas
8. Risk managers are required to forward all information on malpractice and adverse outcomes to the committees that evaluate the competence of medical staff.

Risk management tools

The following tools may be used to identify risk:

1. *Incident reporting* – for example, Nurse Miley attends Mrs Plumb and finds that she has fallen in her room while trying to get into bed. Mrs Plumb tells

Nurse Miley that she is OK, but Nurse Miley alerts the doctor and reports the incident to her supervisor. She is told to fill out an incident report.

2. *Occurrence reporting* – some insurers require organizations to develop a list of adverse patient occurrences that are to be reported by staff; for example, maternal or infant death, the unplanned return of a surgical patient to the hospital or an allergic reaction to medication.

3. *Occurrence screening* – these identify occurrences that are at variance from normal practice, for example the transfer of a patent from a general ward to ICU, nosocomial infections or an unanticipated return to theatres.

The link between risk management and quality assurance

Risk management and quality assurance are two activities that sometimes overlap (Kavaler and Spiegel 2003), as seen in tables 7.1 and 7.2.

Table 7.1 Similarities between risk management and quality assurance

Risk management	Quality assurance
Protects the financial assets of the institution	Demonstrates the organization's caring philosophy
Protects humans and resources	Improves the performance of all staff and protects patients
Protects humans and property	
Reduces loss by focusing on individual loss or accidents	Focuses on the delivery of quality care
Prevents incidents by improving quality of care through monitoring of activities	According to standards and measurable criteria, sets quality of care requirement
	Continuously monitors problem areas to prevent future incidents
Examines each incident using the risk management process:	Searches for non-conformance using quality assurance processes:
• Risk identification	• Problem identification
• Risk analysis	• Problem assessment
• Risk control	• Corrective action
• Risk financing.	• Follow-up
	• Report of findings.

Carroll (2009) in her edited text on healthcare risk management cites the following steps as essential to the risk management process:

1. Identify and analyse loss exposure, for example property, liability, personnel.
2. Consider alternative risk techniques, for example exposure avoidance, loss reduction, segregation of exposure, contractual transfer.

Table 7.2 Differences

Risk management	Quality assurance
Concerned with acceptable levels of care from a legal view	Concerned with best level of care
Focuses on all humans and events	Focuses on patient care
Focuses on legal, insurance and risk financing activities.	Focuses on improving care.

3. Select the best risk (or combination of) management, risk management, technique(s).
4. Implement.
5. Monitor (evaluate) and improve the risk management programme.

As can be seen, Carroll includes areas very similar to those of Kavaler and Spiegel (2003), but she includes evaluation as a key element of risk management.

Key points

- Risk management and quality assurance are different, although some overlap is evident.
- Risk management focuses on financial management.
- Quality assurance focuses on quality of care.

Complaints management

There have been an increasing number of complaints from patients and carers going to litigation over the past decade and the NHS Litigation Authority (NHSLA) state that approximately £470 million has been claimed between 2003 and 2004 (NHSLA 2005). The National Patients Safety Agency (2007) state that preventable harm from medication errors could cost the NHS up to £750 million per year. McSherry and Pearce (2011) attribute these rises to increased

- levels of activity in healthcare organizations
- complexity of treatments
- litigious outlook of patients and carers
- compensation for negligence claims.

However, McSherry and Pearce also state that the vast majority of claims are resolved locally, stressing that openness and honesty, together with robust systems to deal with issues before they become problems, are the main principles to deal with complaints. Organizations need to develop a learning culture supporting employees to report, discuss and learn from incidents and they stress that often complaints arise from systems failure rather than the action of a single member of staff.

McSherry and Pearce present a case study in which a Trust has received a number of complaints from patients (and their carers) who have been admitted to the medical ward following a stroke. The complaints can be divided into poor quality care and poor communication and are illustrated in table 7.3.

Table 7.3 Analysis of complaints

Poor quality care	Poor communication
• Poor attendance to privacy and hygiene needs	• Limited information to patient and carers
• Development of pressure sores	• Inconsistent information from healthcare staff
• Poor attention to nutritional needs	• Failure to disclose information about patient falls
• Limited access to physiotherapy, occupational health and rehabilitation	• Inadequate capture of patient safety data.
• Home assessment and discharge delayed.	

A clinical governance framework supports the organization in understanding and responding to the problem that is distressing patients and carers. In the case outlined above, the process might be

1. Clinical risk identified by letters of complaint, letters acknowledged and investigated by the Complaints Manager
2. Poor quality care identified (poor patient care and poor communication, as above)
3. Review of systems and processes required
4. Clinical audit carried out to explore the nature of the complaint
5. Review of the literature carried out to understand best practice
6. Audit of current process against best practice, identified in point 5 above relating to the risk management process (this may lead to the need for education and training [chapter 5], and recommendations made, implemented and re-audited within 12 months)
7. Review of patient outcomes
8. Leading to a reduction in complaints and a general increase in satisfaction levels.

In the case study given by McSherry and Pearce (2011), the complaints were related to poor systems and processes in which the clinicians had to work, rather than to the clinicians themselves. Following the process above would encourage a review of best Evidence Based Practice against which changes to practice could be made. This would also enable the organization to learn from their mistakes.

The Patients Association issued a report (2013) into complaint handling in NHS Trusts that are signed up to the CARE campaign. The CARE campaign was launched in 2011 and focuses on the four most common complaints notified to their helpline:

1. Poor communication
2. Poor attention to toileting needs
3. Poor attention to nutritional needs
4. Pain relief.

The Complaints Regulations for England (Local Authority Social Services and National Health Service Complaints [England] Regulations 2009) and Wales (NHS Concerns, Complaints and Redress Arrangements [Wales] Regulations 2011) require all Trusts to have systems in place to 'ensure effective, timely and consistent management of complaints' (no page number) and courteous and respectful treatment of complaints. The Care Quality Commission standards of quality and safety and the Ombudsman's principles of good complaint handling also support NHS organizations in the management of complaints. The Patients Associations' Report listed ten criteria that identified good practice in the complaints handling system of the 20 randomly selected Trusts who took part in their research. These are as follows:

1. Criterion 1: A responsible person. Under the Complaints Regulations for England and Wales there is a requirement for a senior member of staff to hold overall responsibility for the management of complaints. This person will be responsible for the complaints management team and a governance committee, both of which will report to the Trust Board regularly.
2. Criterion 2: An exhaustive complaints policy. The Patients Association suggests that the complaints policy of all Trusts should be visible on their websites.
3. Criterion 3: An explanation of the complaints policy in plain language, either on a website or via leaflets.
4. Criteria 4 and 5: Regular reporting to the Trust Board.
5. Criteria 6: Production and publication of regular Complaints reports, ideally on the Trust website.
6. Criterion 7: Production of Annual Reports and Quality Accounts – ideally to be produced by all Trusts.
7. Criterion 8: Staff training – this should also include policy documents on complaints management.
8. Criteria 9 and 10: A culture of and provision for active learning from complaints – this needs to be well developed and at all levels of the organization.

Overview of the main complaints regulations in England and Wales

The NHS Constitution, which sets out the rights and responsibilities of staff and patients sets out some key principles to guide the NHS. Among these are

- the provision of a comprehensive service to all, based on clinical need rather than ability to pay
- a commitment to tax payers, ensuring good value for money
- to be accountable to patients, communities and the public
- to aspire to the highest standards of professionalism and excellence.

In other words, the provision of care that is safe, effective and focused on the experience of the patient.

All NHS, private and third sector providers are legally required to adopt the NHS Constitution in all their dealings with patients, and the rights of complaint and redress are encompassed within this. The Constitution makes the following explicit statements to

- 'the right to have any complaint you make about NHS services dealt with efficiently and to have it properly investigated'
- 'the right to know the outcome of any investigation into your complaint'
- 'the right to take your complaint to the independent Health Service Ombudsman, if you are not satisfied with the way your complaint has been dealt with by the NHS'.
- An updated version of the NHS Constitution (2013) is available on the NHS England website (www.england.nhs.uk) and gives further detail on what patients/carers should expect when making a complaint:
  - Their complaint, whether made verbally, in writing or electronically, will be acknowledged within three working days. The exception to this is where an oral complaint is resolved no later than the next day.
  - They will be offered the opportunity to discuss how their complaint will be handled.
  - They will be informed of the timeframe of when the complaint will be investigated and when they will receive a response.
  - The response will detail the conclusions of the investigation and what actions will be taken as a result of the complaint.

Normally, complaints must be made within 12 months of an issue occurring or within 12 months of the complainant becoming aware that there is an issue. The 2009 regulations also stipulate the requirement for the publicity, monitoring and reporting of complaints (the Local Authority Social Services and National Health Service Complaints (England) Regulations 2009), stating that arrangements for dealing with complaints and how those arrangements may be obtained.

According to the Health and Social Care Act (2008), NHS organizations not only have a legal obligation but also have a contractual obligation and have to be registered with the CQC who ensure that the provision of care meets set standards of quality and safety (CQC 2010). The CQC give 28 outcomes, 16 of which specifically relate to quality and safety of care, clearly stating that each registered body must

- have systems in place to deal with comments and complaints
- support patients/carers to make comments and complaints
- consider, respond and resolve all comments and complaints where possible.

The Parliamentary and Health Service Ombudsman

When a complaint is not resolved locally, it will be directed to the Parliamentary and Health Service Ombudsman for further investigation following the principles described in their Principles of Good Complaint Handling (Parliamentary and Health Service Ombudsman 2009). These are as follows:

1. Getting it right.
2. Being customer focused.
3. Being open and accountable.
4. Acting fairly and proportionately.
5. Putting things right.
6. Seeking continuous improvement.

However, a review in late 2012 (Parliamentary and Health Service Ombudsman 2012) of complaint handling in England showed an 8% rise in complaints highlighting communication problems with complainants. In the period between 2010/11 and 2011/12, the Ombudsman demonstrated 50% more complaints about the NHS, not acknowledging mistakes in care, 13% more complaints about the NHS providing poor explanations to complaints and 42% more complaints about inadequate resolutions.

Activity

The paragraphs above focus on systems in the UK. How does your country/healthcare provider deal with complaints if you do not work in the UK?

- What happens at the local level?
- If not resolved at the local level, how are these complaints resolved?

Serious failings and lessons learnt

We have previously discussed the Mid Staffordshire NHS Foundation Trust, where governance and operational failings of more than a decade resulted in high mortality and complaints were ignored. It was the Healthcare Commission that, in March 2009, highlighted the problems in their investigation into the Trust's high mortality rates for patients admitted as emergencies (Healthcare Commission 2009). Many issues were uncovered, including complaints not being presented to the Trust Board appropriately, and the lack of openness to encourage the discussion and consequent resolution of complaints. They proposed that the following lesson become key to future practice in Trusts:

> Trusts to ensure that systems for governance that appear to be persuasive on paper actually work in practice, and information presented to Boards on performance (including complaints and incidents) is not so summarized that it fails to convey the experience of patients or enable non-executives to scrutinize and challenge on issues relating to patients' care. (Healthcare Commission 2009:11–12)

Furthermore the Commission charged Mid Staffs to improve its quality of care by

- developing and supporting an open learning culture
- collecting accurate information and reporting it appropriately
- investigating and learning from serious incidents such as unexpected death
- ensuring improvements are made following near misses, incidents and complaints
- identifying and reducing risks
- engaging clinicians and developing effective clinical audit
- listening to patients.

These recommendations should be implemented in all healthcare organizations, thereby supporting a strong complaints system as they echo the Heath Service Ombudsman's principles of good complaint handling.

The Healthcare Commission's inquiry prompted an independent inquiry, chaired by Robert Francis, QC, and the inquiry reported in February 2010, revealing neglect and systems failings (including patient experience, staff perceptions and the culture of the Trust) at Mid Staffordshire NHS Foundation Trust. Complaints were supposedly channelled to the Board through the Medical Director and Director of Nursing only but there was little or no evidence of complaints reaching the Chief Executive or the Board. Rather the investigation of complaints was predominantly left at a very local level, that is, staff in the area of the complaint, resulting in defensiveness rather than constructive reporting and learning. The reporting of complaints was slow and did not always address all the issues raised, nor was remedial action implemented. The Francis Inquiry team concluded that '[a] poor complaints system has a negative impact on patents and others who seek to use it. Inadequate responses cause distress and may exacerbate bereavement' (Francis Report 2013:20).

The Francis Inquiry advised the Mid Staffordshire Trust Board to

- ensure adequate responses and plans for resolution of complaints
- ensure that staff are engaged at all levels of the process, that is, from investigation to implementation of lessons learnt
- minimize the risk of the problem occurring again
- make information available on complaints and their resolution to the Board, the governors and the public.

Furthermore, these recommendations would be useful to all Trusts, and, in fact, Recommendation 18 of the Francis Report (2013:28) is 'All NHS trusts and foundation trusts responsible for the provision of hospital services should review their standards, governance and performance in the light of this report.'

Summary

From the above it can be seen that best practice of the management of complaints should include the following:

1. Openness. Trusts must be open and accountable to the public and complaints must be handled thoroughly and transparently.
2. Trusts must have an up-to-date complaints policy, clearly outlining responsibilities, the steps in the complaints handling procedure and the mechanisms in use to report to the Trust Board, for example via the Annual Report, the Complaints Report, etc.
3. The complaints system must be clearly stated on the Trust's website and given in plain English. Leaflets can supplement the use of a website.
4. All complaints must be reported to the Trust Board at each Trust Board meeting, and all documents discussed at the public part of the Board meeting must be available on the website. Additionally, complaints data and trends must be discussed at every Board meeting.
5. Trusts must produce Complaints Reports (including at the least, statistics, trend analysis, lessons learnt and actions taken) and these must be published on their website.
6. Trusts must make public their Annual Reports and Quality Accounts every year.
7. Trusts must invest in staff training in the handling of complaints so that staff are cognizant of the complaints-handling regulations and mechanisms.

8. All complaints must be taken seriously, reported and investigated so that incidents do not reoccur.
9. Trusts must support an open learning culture. Lessons must be learnt following a complaint, complainants must receive a letter detailing what action the Trust has taken together with a later update on the action, each Annual Report, Quality Account and Complaints Report must include a section on actions taken and lessons learnt. All improvements need to be publicized widely.

Additionally, the Patients Association, in their report 'Complaint Handling in NHS Trusts' (2013) signed up to the CARE campaign, and made the following recommendations, which mirror those above:

1. All NHS Trusts must be able to demonstrate that they follow all regulations, obligations and recommendations related to complaints. Trusts without a clear complaints policy must instigate one.
2. All NHS Trusts must be able to demonstrate openness, accountability and transparency in relation to complaints.
3. All NHS Trusts must listen to patients and show respect and understanding rather than defensiveness.
4. Many complaints are due to poor communication. Patients' rights and choices with regard to complaints must be well communicated to them, their carers and their families.
5. The NHS Constitution must be published on all Trust websites as well as on posters throughout the Trust.
6. Information on how to make a complaint must be available on the Trust website, posters and leaflets in the wards and treatment areas.
7. Complaints reports presented at Board meetings must be made available on the Trust website.
8. Complaint related staff-training needs to be identified and made available for all relevant staff.
9. Improvements made after complaints or incidents must be publicized.
10. Best practice is understood, agreed and consistently applied to the Trusts' complaints system.

Key points

- All NHS, private and third sector providers are legally required to adopt the NHS Constitution in all their dealings with patients.
- The rights of complaint and redress are encompassed within the NHS constitution.
- Empowering patients / service users and staff to enable them to shape governance strategies collaboratively (shared governance) will reduce complaints.

Empowering patients/service users and staff to enable them to shape governance strategies collaboratively (shared governance)

Definitions of shared governance are somewhat confusing.

> Shared governance is a journey, not a destination. Organizations pursuing shared governance move incrementally from past orientations where the few rule to an orientation where many learn to make consensual decisions. (Hess 2004: no page number)

But Hess goes on to state that 'Nursing shared governance is hard to define. Its structures and processes are different in every organisation.'

Porter O'Grady (2004) possibly gives a more helpful definition: 'Shared governance is, in short, simply a structural model through which nurses can express and manage their practice with a higher level of professional autonomy' (Porter-O'Grady 2004:251).

The literature suggests that the common characteristics of shared governance include accountability, empowerment, participation and collaboration in decisions that affect patient care, including decisions once held to be the realm of management.

Nurses who are involved in shared governance need to be orientated towards constant change and professional development and also acknowledge the need for a cultural shift in their organization. Additionally, and importantly, Hess (2004: no page number) argues that shared governance should include everyone's voice, including patients': 'Shared governance models that include only nurses can become exclusionary and eventually ineffectual by focusing on the goals of a single profession, instead of the organization as a whole.'

There is increasingly more literature highlighting how patients are included in decision-making, supporting the concept of patients becoming co-designers (as discussed previously in chapter 1) of the delivery of their treatment. Shared decision-making that includes the patient's voice has been associated with improved health outcomes and high patient satisfaction (Edward and Elwyn 2009).

Stigglebout et al. (2012) argue that the most important reason for supporting patients to engage in shared decision-making is one of ethics. Beauchamp and Childress (2001) give four ethical principals and these can be applied to shared decision-making as follows:

- Supporting patients to make reasoned informed choices supports their *autonomy.*
- Supporting patients to make reasoned informed choices supports the concept of *beneficence* by balancing the benefits of treatment against risks and cost, and therefore *non-maleficence* (avoiding harm).

- Supporting patients to make reasoned informed choices supports the concept of *justice* (distributing benefits, risks and costs fairly) as patients usually make more conservative decisions than doctors, and often elect to have fewer procedures.

However, despite these benefits, shared decision-making is far from routine. Stigglebout et al. (2012) suggest the need for a position of 'equipoise' or balance, suggesting to the patient that there is often no best choice, that a decision must be made and that doing nothing is also an option. Patients must be given all the facts and will need statistics to weigh up the pros and cons.

In the past it has been argued that most decision-making was made by well-educated middle-class patients in high-income countries. However, evidence now suggests that providing information in a way that is accessible to patients with lower literacy levels enables them to make informed decisions about their care.

Whatever the aspired goal, shared decision-making requires a cultural shift among healthcare professionals, organizations and patients, but the ultimate goal must be that patients are fully placed at the centre of all decisions pertaining to their health. This is encapsulated in the Salzburg statement on shared decision-making (2011), which calls on clinicians to

- acknowledge that they have an ethical obligation to share important decisions with patients
- motivate two-way communication, which not only gives information but encourages patients to ask questions and thereby offer their preferred method of treatment
- provide accurate information about options, uncertainties, benefits and harms of the treatment options.

Barry and Edgman-Levitan (2012) present eight characteristics of care, from the perspective of patients, and these are

1. Respect for the patient's values, preferences and expressed needs
2. Co-ordinated and integrated care
3. Clear, high-quality information and education for patients, their carers and families
4. Physical comfort, including pain management
5. Emotional support and the reduction of fear and anxiety
6. Involvement of carers, families and friends
7. Continuity of care
8. Access to care.

All of these can be reached if patients and their families are empowered to design, implement and evaluate care systems.

Activity

- Thinking about your place of work, how well are patients supported in making decisions about their treatment?
- Who blocks this process and why?
- How might you be able to support your patients in becoming more autonomous?

Key point

- Patients should be involved in the design, implementation and evaluation of healthcare systems (co-designing – chapter 1).

Key point summary

There are four approaches to quality: quality control, total quality management, quality management and continuous quality improvement. Quality control evaluates, monitors and regulates services provided to consumers. TQM and CQI differ but also have overlapping similarities:

- TQM and CQI both link to the organization's strategic plan, involve education and training and focus on areas for improvement.
- CQI is more likely to refer to the clinical setting, whereas TQM is more industry based.

CQI is a management philosophy and is central to clinical governance. Risk management involves risk identification, risk analysis, risk control and risk financing. Risk management focuses on finances, whereas quality assurance focuses on care, but there are also similarities:

- Both protect the service user.
- They both prevent incidences by continuously monitoring activities.

The four most common complaints are poor communication, poor attention to toileting needs, poor attention to nutritional needs and pain relief. These complaints can be reduced by empowering patients/service users and staff through shared governance (accountability, empowerment, participation and collaboration).

Implications for practice

- It is imperative that staff report 'near misses', as these inform risk management.

- Teams/staff should be involved in risk analysis, so that they understand what happened and why it happened.
- All staff need to know what the complaints procedure is.
- If possible, complaints should firstly be sensitively dealt with at the local level.
- All staff need to be cognizant of the organization's policies pertaining to complaints that cannot be resolved at the local level.

End-of-chapter questions

1. What is the key difference between quality assurance and CQI?
2. What is the difference between clinical risk and risk management?
3. How does a poor complaints system impact on patients, carers and staff?

See the Appendix on page 194 for suggested answers to these questions.

References

Barry MJ and Edgman-Levitan S (2012) Shared decision-making: The pinnacle of patient-centred care. *New England Journal of Medicine*, 366, 780–781

Beauchamp TL and Childress JF (2001) *Principles of biomedical ethics* (5th ed.). Oxford: Oxford University Press

Care Quality Commission (2010) *Guidance about compliance: Summary of regulations, outcomes and judgement framework.* Available at http://www.cqc.org.uk/sites/default/files/media/documents/guidance_about_compliance_summary.pdf (accessed 10.10.13).

Carroll R (2009) *Risk management handbook for healthcare organizations.* San Francisco: Jossey-Bass

Chandraharan E and Arulkumaran S (2007) Clinical governance. *Obstetrics, Gynaecology and Reproductive Medicine*, 17, 222–224

Cottee C and Harding K (2008) Risk management in obstetrics. *Obstetrics, Gynaecology and Reproductive Medicine*, 18, 155–162

Department of Health (2000) *An organisation with a memory.* London: Department of Health

Department of Health (2004) *National standards, location action. Health and social care standards and planning framework 005/2007I.* Leeds: Department of Health

Edward A and Elwyn G (eds.) (2009) *Shared decision-making in healthcare: Achieving evidence-based patient choice* (2nd ed.). Oxford: Oxford University Press

Feigenbaum AV (1983) *Total quality control.* New York: McGraw-Hill

Fenn P and Egan T (2012) Risk management in the NHS: governance, finance and clinical risk. *Clinical Medicine*, 12 (1), 25–28

Francis Report (2013) *Report of the Mid Staffordshire NHS Trust Foundation Trust Public Inquiry.* London: HMSO

Healthcare Commission (2009) *Investigation into Mid Staffordshire NHS Foundation Trust: Summary report*. Available at http://www.midstaffspublicinquiry.com/key-documents (accessed 30.10.2013)

Hess RG (2004) From bedside to boardroom – nursing shared governance. *Online Journal of Issues in Nursing*, 9 (1). Available at www.nursingworld.org/MainMenu-Categories/ANAMarketplace/ANAPeriodicals/OJIN/TableOfContents/Volume92004/No1Jan04/FromBedside to Boardroom.aspx (accessed 18.11.13)

Kavaler F and Spiegel A (2003) *Risk Management in healthcare institutions: A strategic approach* (2nd ed.). Mississauga: Jones and Bartlett

Local Authority Social Services and National Health Service Complaints (England) Regulations (2009) http://www.gov.uk (accessed 21.01.2014)

McLaughlin CP and Kaluzny AD (2006) *Continuous quality improvement in healthcare: Theory, implementations and applications* (3rd ed.). London: Jones and Bartlett

McSherry R and Pearce P (2011) *Clinical Governance: A guide to implementation for healthcare professionals* (3rd ed.). Oxford: Wiley-Blackwell

Mitra A (2012) *Fundamentals of quality control and improvement*. Hoboken: Wiley

NHS Constitution (2013) http://www.england.nhs.uk/2013/03/26/nhs-constitution/ (accessed 30.10.2013)

Parliamentary and Health Service Ombudsman (2009) *Principles of good complaint handling*. Available at http://www.ombudsman.org.uk/improving-public-service/ombudsmansprinciples/principles-of-good-complaint-handling-full (accessed 30.10.2013)

Parliamentary and Health Service Ombudsman (2012) *Listening and learning: The Ombudsman's review of complaint handling in the NHS in England 2011–2012*. Available at http://www.ombudsman.org.uk/__data/assets/pdf_file/0018/18126/FINAL_Listening_and_Learning_NHS_report_2011 12optimised.pdf (accessed 30.10.2013)

Porter-O'Grady T (2004) Overview and summary. Shared governance: Is it a mode for nurses to gain control over their practice? *Online Journal of Issues of Nursing*, 9 (1). Available at www.nursingworld.org/MainMenuCategories/ANAMarketplace/ANAPeriodicals/OJIN/TableOfContents/Volume92004/No1Jan04/Overview.aspx (accessed 18.11.2013)

Salzburg statement on shared decision-making (2011). *British Medical Journal*. Available at http://dx.doi.org/10.1126.bmj.d1745 (accessed 20.1.14)

Smith DG and Wheeler JRC (1992) Strategies and structures for hospital risk management programs. *Healthcare Management Review*, 17 (3), 9–17

Som C (2004) Clinical governance: A fresh look at its definition. *Clinical Governance: An International Journal*, 9, 87–90

Stigglebout AM, Van der Weijden T, De Wit MPT, Frosch D, Legare F, Montori VM, Trevana L and Elwyn G (2012) Shared decision-making: Really putting patients at the centre of healthcare. *British Medical Journal*. Available at http://dx.doi.org/10.1136/bmj.e256

The CARE Campaign (2011) http:/www.thecarecampaign.co.uk/ (accessed 30.10.2013)

The Health and Social Care Act 2008 (Regulated Activities) Regulations 2010. Available at http://www.cqc.org.uk/sites/default/files/media/documents/health_and_social_care_act_2008_regulated_activities.pdf. (accessed 30.10.2013)

The Local Authority Social Services and National Health Service Complaints (England) Regulations (2009). Available at http://www.legislation.gov.uk/uksi/2009/309/regulation/4/made. (accessed 30.10.2013)

The National Health Service (Concerns, Complaints and Redress Arrangements) (Wales), Regulations 2011. Available at http://www.legislation.gov.uk/wsi/2011/704/pdfs/wsi_20110704_mi.pdf. (accessed 30.10.2013)

The Patients Association (2013) Complaint handling in NHS Trusts signed up to the CARE campaign: Reality criteria and identification of best practice. Available at http://www.patients-association.com/Portals/0/Complaint%20handling%20in%20NHS%20Trusts%20signed%20up%20to%20the%20CARE%20campaign_Jan_2013.pdf. (accessed 30.10.2013)

8

Evaluating quality care through audit

Mary Gottwald and Gail E Lansdown

Learning objectives

By the end of this chapter, the reader will be better able to

- identify the rationale for clinical audit
- apply the audit cycle to practice
- recognize barriers to clinical audit
- recognize criteria for successful audit.

Introduction

Clinical audit is an integral part of clinical governance and a key component of the process. It is one of the seven pillars of clinical governance; clinical effectiveness, risk management, education and training, patient and public involvement, staffing and staff management and using information and IT being the other six.

Chapter 1 highlighted a number of high-profile cases in the UK that led to public inquiries focusing on the failure of the NHS. The outcome of these inquiries led to a loss of trust in the NHS. Chapter 2 went on to discuss some examples where the quality of care could be called into question. Chapter 6 focused on the importance of EBP and this chapter will focus on how audit can be used to identify where there is a lack of quality care but also provide evidence for excellent care provision. However, it is important to recognize that EBP and audit have different functions.

Audit is used to support and evaluate continuous quality improvement programmes that are a requirement of all NHS organizations and therefore can lead to a reduction in high-profile cases (NICE 2002). The significance of these quality improvement programmes is to regain public trust in healthcare services.

Audit versus research

Audit measures practice against standards and performance. Audit poses the question 'Are we doing the right thing in the right way'? Research, on the other hand, asks the question 'What is the right thing to do'? Table 8.1 highlights the difference between audit and research.

Clinical audit

In the UK the key aim of the Darzi report (2008) (chapter 1) is to improve the quality of care through the management of risk reduction. Results from clinical audits can identify these improvements as well as identify any reasons for lack of improvement. Audit can be used to 'benchmark' organizations in relation to similar organizations. This could result in extra demands and pressures being imposed on teams to improve, but on the other hand can be motivating for staff if a 'gold standard' is achieved (Paskins et al. 2010:204).

Clinical audit is not a new concept and over time healthcare organizations have been scrutinized both internally and externally. Consequently audit is now adopted by all health and social care professions who have a duty to conform to audit processes (Cowan 2002, Sale 2005, Clouston and Westcott 2005,

Table 8.1 The difference between audit and research

Research	Audit
Generates new knowledge	Current knowledge is used to best
Is initiated by researchers	effect
Is theory driven (hypothesis based)	Usually led by service providers
Is often a one-off event	Is practice based (standard based)
Is large scale for prolonged periods of	Is an ongoing process
time	Usually less large scale and prolonged
Often involves statistical analysis	than research
May involve randomly allocating service	Minimal statistical analysis
users to different treatment groups	Never involves randomly allocating
May involve administration of placebo	service users to treatment groups
Often requires approval from an ethical	Never involves placebos
committee	Never requires approval from ethical
	committees

(Adapted from Dilnawaz et al. 2012)

Benjamin 2008). Audit is a quality improvement process that was first introduced to the NHS by the 1989 White Paper 'Working for Patients' (Department of Health 1989), becoming a mandatory component for all hospital doctors as of 1998 (Department of Health 1998).

According to NICE (2002:viii), clinical audit 'should be at the very heart of clinical governance systems'. In recent times there has been a move away from 'optional' clinical audit activity to a more 'obligatory' approach and hence clinical audit has become a pillar and formal part of the clinical governance framework in the UK and elsewhere in the world. Chapter 5 presented the case for continued professional development (CPD) and because auditing clinical practice highlights areas of both good and poor practice, it enables professionals continuously to pursue best Evidence Based Practice (chapter 6).

The public inquiries discussed in chapter 1 will all have included an audit of the healthcare provision and will have identified recommendations, some of which will link to audit. For example, the Bristol Royal Infirmary Inquiry (2001:167) identified 198 recommendations, three of which are specific to audit:

Recommendation 143: Audit should be central to organizational monitoring systems and processes.

Recommendation 144 therefore must be supported by healthcare Trusts so that staff are provided with necessary resources to carry out an audit.

Recommendation 145: Clinical staff contracts therefore stipulated the requirement to participate in audit.

It is therefore imperative that staff understand what an 'audit' involves. NICE (2002:1) provide a clear definition of this:

> Clinical audit is a quality improvement process that seeks to improve patient care and outcomes through systematic review of care against explicit criteria and the implementation of change. Aspects of the structure, processes, and outcomes of care are selected and systematically evaluated against explicit criteria. Where indicated changes are implemented at an individual, team or service level and further monitoring is used to confirm improvement in healthcare delivery.

As can be seen in this definition, audit is a quality improvement and a change process based on the appraisal of current practice.

Donebedian (1966) suggested three aspects of performance: structure (what is needed), process (what is done) and outcome of care (what is expected). Audit usually falls into one of these, or may include two or more.

Examples of each of these are given in table 8.2.

Table 8.2 Structure, process and outcome audit

Structure	This relates to the resources that are considered essential so that organizations meet their strategic objectives, and will include aspects such as amenities, equipment, staffing and skill mix.
Process	This links to practice: clinical decision-making, assessment, prescribing, clinical interventions such as surgery, physiotherapy, occupational therapy and methods of record keeping.
Outcome	Outcome audit is linked to process audit and concerns the expected short- and long-term impact of healthcare provision. For example, the short-term impact of prescribing statins (process) to reduce cholesterol levels, will impact on the likelihood (outcome) of not having a heart attack or stroke in the long term.

(NICE 2002, Wright and Hill 2003, Benjamin 2008, Donnellon et al. 2013)

Audit involves examination of processes employed in healthcare to ensure that procedures are followed, standards achieved, no impropriety occurs, stakeholders are optimally treated and best value is obtained from the resources consumed (Sale 2005). Audit involves measuring 'current practice' against 'best practice': comparing what is being done against what should be done. Relevant changes required to improve the quality of care can be implemented and then re-audited to measure the final outcomes (Clouston and Westcott 2005:146). Audit is not just about identifying poor practice but also about identifying examples of good high-quality practice. It is important for teams to understand why practice is considered good, and conversely why some practices are considered less than good (Wright and Hill 2003, Sale 2005).

If the results of audit do identify poor practice, then education and training at the team level (chapter 5) becomes important, for example workshops on clinical guidelines, processes of care, could be covered within workshops (Wright and Hill 2003). Audit results can be influential in that they can lead to organizations reviewing and changing practice (Paskins et al. 2010). However, as already identified in chapter 4, changing practice is not always easy and therefore good leadership and teamwork are required.

It is important to be aware that clinical audit has a 'mixed' reception amongst healthcare professionals and some government publications – 'Good Doctors, Safer Patients' (Department of Health 2006) and the 'Assurance and Safety' White Paper (Department of Health 2007) concluded that clinical audit was falling short of its potential and thus needed to be strengthened.

NICE (2002) stipulates that for audit to be successful the environment needs to be supportive and the methods used need to enable staff to engage in audit projects that enhance the provision of quality healthcare. If we return to the Department of Health's (1998:33) definition of clinical governance, we can see the importance of organizations creating supportive environments: 'A framework through which organisations are accountable for continuously improving the quality of services and safeguarding high standards of care by creating an environment in which clinical care will flourish.'

Audit will not be successful if changes to practice are not implemented and the quality of services improved (Pickering and Thompson 2003).

Central principles of audit

The previous chapter 6 focused on Evidence Based Practice (EBP), and one tool that has been effective in supporting EBP is clinical audit. Audit sits in the fifth and final stage of the evidence cycle (Morrell and Harvey 1999):

1. Formulating a clinical question (using PICO)
2. Finding the evidence (searching the research literature)
3. Critiquing the evidence (using a critiquing framework)
4. Using the evidence to bring about change
5. Evaluate using audit.

Morrell and Harvey (1999) list the central principles of audit as

1. Professionally led
2. An educational process
3. A routine part of clinical practice
4. Based on the setting of standards
5. Generating results that can be used to improve the quality of care
6. Involving management in both process and outcome
7. Confidential at both the clinician and patient level
8. Being informed by the views of both clinicians and patients.

Furthermore, audit is central to clinical governance, which is illustrated in figure 8.1.

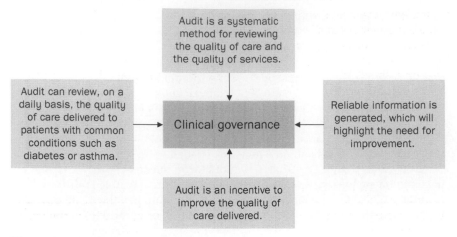

Figure 8.1 Linking audit to clinical governance.

As can be seen, clinical audit is a quality improvement process that aims to improve patient care by systematically reviewing care against explicit criteria, leading to the implementation of change if necessary.

Designing audit

Chambers and Wakley (2005) suggest that the audit cycle has nine steps, three of which will be considered here. The remaining steps will be considered under the audit cycle.

Working with others, prioritizing and selecting the audit topic

In order to engage healthcare professionals in audit there need to be perceived benefits. The benefits may be to patients, colleagues, the organization or the NHS. An audit topic is therefore likely to focus on an area that is

1. High risk or
2. High volume or
3. Causes concern or
4. High cost.

If the audit focuses on a process or system, then the benefits would need to have a bearing on efficiency or effectiveness. The outcome of all audits must have the potential to support improvements.

Chambers and Wakley (2005) suggest that the normal audit categories are

- the frequency or volume of a service
- risks associated with the provision of care

- problems associated with the provision of care
- the effectiveness of the delivery of care
- the cost of delivering care.

It is also important to remember that audit usually involves change and that communication is key.

As discussed earlier, audit may focus on structure, process or outcome or a mixture of all three. Chambers and Wakley (2005) suggest an audit protocol (table 8.3) that encapsulates all the stages of audit.

Table 8.3 Audit stages and protocol

1. Choose a topic that is a priority for you or your team or the NHS in general. What is it?

2. What problem are you addressing?

3. How did you choose this topic (tick all that apply):
   - In discussion with colleagues
   - Decided on behalf of work colleagues
   - It was requested by another team
   - It is part of the Trust's business plan
   - It is part of the Trust's strategic plan
   - Patient or carer request
   - Other

4. Why did you choose the topic? Is it a priority?
   If yes, for whom is it a priority?
   - The government?
   - Your Trust or organization?
   - The team?
   - Patients?
   - Yourself?
   - The profession?
   - A National Service Framework? If yes, which one?
   - A NICE requirement?
   - A previous or recent adverse event?

5. Is the topic important? If yes, is it
   - High cost?
   - A common problem?
   - Life threatening?
   - Related to your local population?
   - A routine check of every day care or service provision?
   - An example of inadequate care?
   What other reasons are important?

(continued)

Table 8.3 (*Continued*)

6. What are your objectives? Are they SMART?

7. Have you designed your audit protocol in such a way that everyone knows who is doing what, why, when and how?

8. What principles of good practice are included in your audit?
   - It has multidisciplinary input
   - It involves colleagues as appropriate
   - It considers relevant interfaces, for example how and where you work with other NHS professionals, the non-health section and care settings
   - It incorporates the views of carers and patients in training, planning, monitoring and delivery
   - It is capable of achieving health gains
   - Input and commitment from managers/the organization is incorporated

9. Who will lead the audit?

10. Who else will be involved?

11. What resources do you need, for example training, resources, facilities, skills, people and time?

12. What criteria have you selected and why?

13. What standards have you selected? From where did they originate?

14. What data/information will you gather as a baseline?

15. When will you start? What is the timetable?

16. What system do you have for reviewing the results of the audit and reviewing performance against the agreed standards? Who will decide and who will make any necessary changes?

17. What changes do you hope to make?

18. Are these changes possible within current resources and skills? If necessary, from where will you obtain additional resources?

19. Are you being realistic in expecting change?

20. What interventions or changes in service or practice will you introduce if your performance does not reach the standards you have set? What resources will you need for these interventions/changes?

21. What specific outcomes do you expect from introducing the intervention or change?

22. How will you measure these?

23. How will you demonstrate any improvements or changes from the baseline arising from the intervention(s)?

24. When and how will you re-audit your improved or changed practice or service?

(Adapted from Chambers and Wakley 2005:18 and reproduced with permission)

Examining the literature and setting reasonable standards based on the literature

Having defined a quality issue, it is important to interrogate the literature in a systematic way to find research articles that will address this issue. Readers are referred to chapter 6 where this has been discussed in depth. Having a clear understanding of the evidence enables practitioners to then set standards against which to monitor their practice.

Designing the audit: audit tools

The nursing profession was the first to implement standard-setting in the 1980s and therefore led the field in a systematic approach to monitoring quality against standards. Sale (2005:199) describes a number of, as she calls them, 'off-the-shelf' tried and tested nursing audit tools. Three of the most commonly used are Qualpacs (Wandelt and Ager 1974), Phaneuf's Nursing Audit (Phaneuf 1976) and Monitor (Goldstone et al. 1983).

Qualpacs

Qualpacs (Quality Patient Care Scale) is an American tool and measures the quality of care received by the patient from the ward or unit nursing staff. Consisting of 68 items, it measures the direct and indirect interaction of nursing staff with patients and is divided into six categories:

1. Psychosocial (individual): 15 items
2. Psychosocial (group): 8 items
3. Physical: 15 items
4. General: 15 items
5. Communication: 8 items
6. Professional implications: seven items.

Each item supplies prompts to assist in completing the audit, for example under Psychological (Individual), the first item is 'Patient receives nurse's full attention'. The prompts are as follows:

- The patient is appropriately responded to verbally and non-verbally, without being asked to repeat phrases.
- Staff assume positions that will aid in observation and communication with patient.
- Conversation of staff is restricted to the patient who is receiving care.
- And so on.

The prompts may be amended to suit the situation, as it is the item that is scored and not the prompt. Table 8.4 lists the advantages and disadvantages of Qualpac.

Table 8.4 Advantages and disadvantages of Qualpac

Advantages:
Rigorously tested and therefore reliable and valid;
Has been used in the UK, in the Nursing Development Unit in Oxford;
Data are provided by direct observation;
Uses more than one method of concurrent review;
By evaluating performance, provides nurses with an insight into their practice,
    thus improving patient care;
Provides positive feedback to individuals and the team.

Disadvantages:
The values are American;
Highly skilled and trained observers required;
Is time consuming, both to administer and score;
Observer bias can occur if observer is influenced by their own attitudes and
    expectations;
May be subjective as relies on the professional judgement of the observer.

(Sale 2005:205)

Phaneuf's nursing audit

This is a retrospective audit of the patient's records based on the assumption that good notes reflect good care. Using the seven functions of nursing developed by Lesnik and Anderson (1955), Phaneuf designed 50 components to enable auditors to evaluate the quality of care from the medical records.

An audit committee with a minimum of five members will audit no more than ten patients per month, with each audit taking approximately 15 minutes. Auditors will require training. As with Qualpac, this audit tool also has advantages and disadvantages which can be seen in table 8.5.

Monitor

Based on the Rush Medicus methodology (developed in Chicago between 1972 and 1975), Monitor was designed by North-West Region and Newcastle-upon-Tyne Polytechnic. A conceptual framework was developed to measure the nursing process, and patient needs and criteria were developed to evaluate quality of care within this framework. Six objectives representing the nursing process were identified:

1. A nursing plan is formulated.
2. The physical needs of the patient are met.
3. The physical, emotional and social needs of the patient are met.
4. Achievement of nursing care objectives is evaluated.
5. Unit procedures are followed for the protection of all patients.
6. The delivery of nursing care is facilitated by administrative and managerial services.

Table 8.5 Advantages and disadvantages of Phaneuf's nursing audit

Advantages:
It can be used in all areas of nursing;
The seven functions are easily understood;
Scoring is reasonably simple;
The results are easy to understand;
It assesses all those involved in recording care;
It is useful if accurate records of care are kept.

Disadvantages:
Having been devised in the USA, it does not take account of British nursing,
    policies, politics and procedures;
It cannot be used in areas where the nursing process has not been implemented;
It is time-consuming;
Auditors need to be trained;
It only evaluates record keeping and therefore helps to improve documentation
    rather than the delivery of care;
Based on assumptions – good records denote good care and what is done is
    documented and what is documented is done.

(Sale 2005:211)

Table 8.6 Advantages and disadvantages of Monitor

Advantages:
Information is collected from many areas including documentation systems,
    management systems, the environment, delivery of care and outcomes.
It gives feedback on quality of care.
It improves the performance of staff.
It gives an indication of patient satisfaction.
It can compare performance across wards and Trusts.
It measures the effectiveness of the nursing process.
It provides information that can be used in the future planning of training and
    development.

Disadvantages:
Trained observers are required and this has a resource implication.
It requires the purchase of several copies of the document.
As the criteria are preset, there is no ownership of the process by the staff who
    are being measured.
There is no clear statement on its philosophy of nursing.
There are problems with observer reliability and subjectivity. This could be
    reduced with extensive training.

(Sale 2005: 217)

Each of the six objectives contain a number of subobjectives, and criteria were developed so that yes, no or not applicable answers may be given. As with the two other audit tools discussed above, there are also advantages and disadvantages to Monitor (table 8.6).

These are three of a number of 'off-the-shelf' tools to audit the nursing process. They have their advantages and their disadvantages, one of the main advantages being that it can take a great deal of time to develop a good audit tool. However, the focus of these three tools is somewhat non-specific as they cover a wide range of criteria.

Not all audits require a validated tool as discussed above, and teams may choose to design the audit process themselves. This being the case, Chambers and Wakley's (2005) suggested audit protocol may be helpful (table 8.3).

The audit cycle

Having chosen a relevant tool or designed an audit tool, the next stage is to carry out the audit. In order for quality improvement programmes to be successful, the process of audit needs to be continuous and cyclical and as illustrated in figure 8.2. At the local level, once standards have

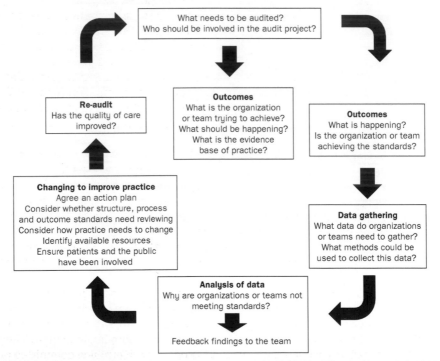

Figure 8.2 The audit cycle. (Adapted from NICE 2002, Wright and Hill 2003 and Benjamin 2008)

been met teams need to re-audit, set higher standards and improve the level of quality further. At a more extensive level the audit process may involve healthcare services within a specific region or nationally within the country.

Each stage of the audit cycle illustrated in figure 8.2 will now be discussed in more depth.

Stage 1: What needs to be audited and who needs to be involved?

Clinical audit is the method used to evaluate performance against evidence-based standards. So the aspect of audit that needs to be considered should be on a quality issue where there is good evidence available on what comprises good quality care. For example, evidence available in relation to treatment and prevention of pressure ulcers, hospital acquired infections or medication errors (see activity box below). If this evidence is limited, then teams will find it difficult to identify standards that ensure best practice (Wright and Hill 2003, McSherry and Pearce 2011). The clinical aspect chosen for audit should also link to national priorities such as the UK National Service Framework standards of care (Swage 2004).

Organizations will have a clinical audit lead who will need to work along-side everybody who is involved in patient care, such as, health and social care professionals, stakeholders, service users and patients. Everyone involved with either delivering or experiencing healthcare needs to be included in dis-cussions related to which aspects of clinical practice ought to be audited. As well as involving relevant individuals in discussions, auditors can gather data through records of complaints (chapter 7), risk management data (chapter 7), significant events ('near misses'), patient satisfaction surveys, interviews (NICE 2002, Pickering and Thompson 2003) or through the Patient Voices Pro-gramme (chapter 1).

If there have been a number of complaints, for example in relation to long waiting times in the Accident and Emergency department, the teams may choose to carry out an audit so that causes can be identified. This could also involve setting up a quality circle where stakeholders, patients and service users can be included and/or teams can use the fishbone analy-sis to identify causes of poor quality care (chapter 3). Swage (2004) recom-mends that stakeholders be included in the discussions on which quality issues to audit and suggests that they may well also be involved in the audit process.

As well as choosing topics that link to the evidence base of practice, topics need to link to the strategic objectives and organizational priorities (Benjamin 2008). Organizations and teams may carry out significant events analysis, which could lead to the decision for a clinical audit being implemented. They will have to prioritize and it may be that the clinical governance committee or quality improvement committee makes the final decisions on which aspects of clinical practice will undergo clinical audit (NICE 2002).

Activity

Explore the following links (accessed 05.11.2013):

* http://www.thecochranelibrary.com/view/0/index.html
* http://www.nice.org.uk
* http://www.evidence.nhs.uk

These links will identify literature and evidence-based guidelines, for example Pressure Ulcers CG29 (2001). Practice can then be compared with standard statements in the guidelines.

Activity

Explore the following links, where you can access videos illustrating real-life patient experiences:

* http://healthtalkonline.org
* http://healthtalkonline.org/young-peoples-experiences

Stage 2: Outcomes

In order to meet the outcomes, organizations and teams need to have identified measurable standards. These audit criteria are explicit statements that define an outcome that can be measured. They should relate to important aspects of care and be derived from the best available evidence. Having explicit selection criteria will ensure that the data collected is precise and that only essential information is gathered.

Standards should relate to important standards that are thresholds of the expected compliance for each criterion; they should be based on the best evidence available. A minimum standard describes the lowest acceptable standard of performance and is often used as the 'cut-off' for acceptable and unacceptable performance. 'Ideal standards describe the care it should be possible to give under ideal conditions, with no constraints' (Anderson, cited in Benjamin 2008:1244). Unfortunately such standards cannot usually be achieved. Whilst most people would like to see ideal standards – and many audit teams write such standards – in the 'real world' of healthcare in the twenty-first century they may be unrealistic. The development of standards will usually involve a combination of clinical experience and a review of the available evidence.

In order to understand whether these standards are being achieved within realistic timeframes set, there is a requisite that standards be monitored. Sale (2005:54) posits that there is a difference between the monitoring of standards and auditing standards. Monitoring standards identifies any gaps and provides teams with a 'snapshot' of whether quality care is being provided because the standards have been met. A 'detailed portrait' and clinical audit are required when there are unmet aspects of the standards.

Activity

Explore the following links (accessed 05.11.2013), which identify the various National Service Frameworks and expected standards:

* http://www.wales.nhs.uk/sites3/home.cfm?orgid=334
* http://www.nhs.uk/nhsengland/nsf/Pages/Nationalserviceframeworks.aspx
* https://www.gov.uk/government/publications/quality-standards-for-mental-health-services
* http://www.sign.ac.uk

Stage 3: Data gathering

Data is in the main gathered through examining patient case records, and therefore ethical principles such as anonymity and confidentiality must be respected (Swage 2004). Wright and Hill (2003:103) make three suggestions that help this process:

1. *Define and agree what information is required*: In relation to auditing the quality of care, data on 'diagnosis, co-morbidity, interventions and complications' would be valuable.
2. *Design and pilot an audit proforma*: It is important to carry out a pilot to ensure the data is relevant and easy to analyse (Hicks 2004).
3. *Select the sample*: Avoiding bias within audit is crucial and therefore sampling methods should either (a) include all patient records within a given time period or (b) include a random sample, for example using random number tables (Hicks 2004). The sample selected should be one that reflects the characteristics of the population from which it has been drawn. Data collected may be retrospective, concurrent or prospective. The differences between these are highlighted in table 8.7.

Table 8.7 Data collection

Categories	Retrospective	Prospective	Concurrent
Definition	Data collected by looking back over practice; i.e patients have been discharged.	Data collected from this point onwards, starting at a future date. In the future either a retrospective or concurrent audit will be carried out.	Data are collected on patients who are still in hospital or receiving care, and so the audit is concurrent with actual patient care.
When to use	When looking at what has happened in a chosen topic area.	Data currently not available; data of poor quality.	When patients care plans need to be reviewed.
Advantages	Can be faster; provides a baseline.	Avoids using poor data; allows design of clear data collection.	The patient benefits at the time of the audit because problems are identified at the time of care.
Disadvantages	Past service users do not benefit.	No baseline provided; can be time consuming.	Time consuming and costly to implement.

(Hicks 2004 and Dilnawaz et al. 2012)

Activity

If you are going to lead an audit project, the following questions will be useful to consider:

- Who is going to collect the data?
- How is the data going to be collected?
- Who will develop the data collection proforma?
- Who will pilot the proforma and amend if needed?

Stage 4: Analysis of data

Once data have been collected, they need to be compared with the standards and criteria set and the evidence base of practice as identified by agreed national standards, such as the UK National Service Frameworks or NICE guidelines. Following the analysis, the findings must be disseminated to the team.

Standards could include a reduction in errors such as medication errors, hospital acquired infections or pressure ulcers and standard statements may be written as follows:

- By the end of 2015, there will be a 40% reduction in medication errors.

The analysis of data can result in both positive and negative outcomes, for example if a 60% reduction in medication errors has been achieved, then this demonstrates a clear improvement in patient care. On the other hand, if a 35% reduction was identified, this conveys a need to continue to focus on improving processes such as the prescription of medication. When setting standards, it is important to consider the percentage, because setting a standard too high (100%) may not be realistic or achievable for the organization and therefore setting an optimum standard is required. Once the standard of 40% has been achieved, a higher percentage can be agreed.

Stage 5: Changing practice to improve the quality of care

This can be the most challenging part of the audit cycle because the results of the data analysis are likely to require a change in practice and, as discussed in chapter 4, this can be a difficult experience for practitioners. Once areas of poor practice have been identified, discussions can take place on how to manage individual or team poor performance (Donnellon et al. 2013). Donnellon et al. (2013) suggest that if formative feedback is provided to individuals or teams that encourages reflection on practice and if support is provided that will facilitate the development of their knowledge, skills and clinical decision-making, then this can only enhance practice. CPD programmes (chapter 5) are an important aspect of changing practice. Agreeing an action plan will facilitate changes to practice and will enable teams to monitor progress in relation to agreed objectives, strategies and actions. The action plan needs to include SMART objectives, the tasks, and who is responsible for each task.

Stage 6: Re-audit

The last stage of the audit cycle involves repeating the audit. This audit must be carried out in the same way as the initial audit to ensure that accurate and valid comparisons can be made. The results from the re-audit will identify whether changes have been made and the quality of healthcare provision improved. Re-auditing can also demonstrate whether there is an increasing trend in meeting required standards (Donnellon et al. 2013, Swage 2004). It may then be necessary to agree further changes and another audit at a later date.

Advantages, disadvantages and barriers to clinical audit

Advantages and disadvantages

In order to review the benefits and disadvantages of clinical audit, Johnston et al. (2000) carried out a systematic review of articles retrieved from Medline and CINAHL databases for the years 1992 to 1997. A total of 93 articles were reviewed, across a range of audit processes, including individual audit projects, retrospective reviews of department audit programmes at the interface between primary and secondary care. The experiences of all staff grades, from medical consultants to professionals allied to medicine and from those involved in both uniprofessional and multiprofessional care, were collected. A summary of the findings is shown below.

Advantages

* Improved communication across clinical groups
* Improved patient care
* Increased professional satisfaction
* Improved administration

Disadvantages

* Reduced clinical ownership
* Fear of litigation
* Professional isolation
* Suspicions due to hierarchy and territorialism

Garg et al. (2010:49) also identify some benefits for the auditor. Carrying out an audit provides staff with a chance to develop their 'skills in project management, team-working, reflective practice, clinical governance and service development'.

Barriers

Whilst having discussed the benefits of a clinical audit, there are a number of barriers to implementing it in the workplace. Chambers and Wakley (2005) give the following barriers to audit:

* negative attitudes and an unwillingness to participate
* willingness of the whole team to be involved (taking a multidisciplinary approach)
* audit is seen as an extra undertaking
* overwhelmed healthcare practitioners feel they have insufficient time
* lack of resources, especially time

- lack of training in audit and evidence-based skills
- patients and service users unwilling to take part
- lack of communication
- imbalance between an individual's desire to audit and the needs of the service
- failure to provide a supportive climate for audit, and sensitivity as some individuals may feel uncomfortable that their performance is being monitored
- fear of and resistance to change
- failure to complete the audit cycle
- the cost of carrying out audit and implementing change

Activity

- Think of the last time you were involved in an audit. Did any of the barriers listed above impede the process?

Johnston et al. (2000) surmised that there were five main barriers to clinical audit:

1. Lack of resources
2. Lack of expertise/advice in design and analysis
3. Difficulties between groups and group members
4. Lack of an overall plan for audit
5. Organizational hindrance

Balancing these, Johnston et al. (2000) found the key factors supporting audit to be

1. Modern medical records systems
2. Effective training
3. Motivated and dedicated staff
4. Good leadership
5. Protected time
6. Dialogue between purchasers and providers
7. Mechanisms to support data collection, including IT systems
8. Strategy and planning
9. High levels of audit activity with monitoring and reporting as integral to the process
10. Protective time for clinicians
11. A supportive organization.

Activity

- Bearing in mind that this article was published in 2000, which, if any of the disadvantages and barriers still exist in your place of work?

The recommendation of Johnston et al. (2000) to seek the opinions of clinicians on the process of a new audit was picked up by Paskins and colleagues in 2010. Examining an annual regional rheumatology audit that has been running in the West Midlands since 2000, they found that this was viewed to be an efficient use of resources and had unexpected educational benefits whilst promoting good relationships across the region.

Garg et al. (2010) focused their research on why staff do not become engaged in the audit process. They identified some of the difficulties and barriers trainee doctors experienced when carrying out clinical audit, and these are illustrated in table 8.8. This National UK study involved an online survey using a questionnaire that was disseminated to student doctors working within psychiatry. Responding to this survey were 504 doctors, who gave a response rate of 89%; this response rate is high and therefore results can be deemed to be relevant (Denscombe 2010). Altogether these participants had been involved with 2267 audits. However, the completion rate of the audit cycle, in particular completion of stage 6 as discussed above, was considered low.

Table 8.8 Barriers to getting involved in clinical audit

Time	Work based pressures on top of routine clinical activities impacted on available time to carry out an audit. Examples cited included time taken to attend CPD courses, time to study for exams and time to complete job applications and attend for interviews. Time was not specifically allocated for the audit and so had to be carried out within rostered clinical hours and often trainee doctors were not in placement long enough to complete the audit cycle.
Lack of support	Lack of training to carry out an audit. Lack of support from medical records departments in providing information. Absence of management, senior clinicians and clinical governance team members at audit meetings.
Lack of motivation	Respondents identified that if team members disagreed with the audit findings, were resistant to changing practice following the outcome of the audit or if recommendations were not implemented, then the auditors lost motivation to carry out further audits.
Poor communication	Poor communication leading to conflict within teams prevented changes to practice being carried forward. Results of audits were not always clearly disseminated and therefore teams were not aware of the impact of changing practice on improved quality of patient care.

(Garg et al. 2010:48)

Activity

Compare the findings of Chalmers and Wakley (2005) to those of Garg et al. (2010). Bearing in mind that these authors were writing five years apart, what reduction in barriers, if any, can you see?

Approaches to audit

Having discussed the aspects that need to be considered when designing an audit tool, the audit cycle, barriers to audit and the strengths and limitations of audit, table 8.9 illustrates a number of approaches to audit that teams and individuals will need to consider.

Table 8.9 Approaches to audit

Self-audit	Using the evidence (as discussed in chapter 6) to ensure practice is up to date and evidence based
Peer audit	Asking a colleague to observe practice to ensure that it meets set standards
Critical incident audit	The multidisciplinary team discusses anonymous cases that have either caused concern or had an unexpected outcome
Supervisory audit	Often undertaken as part of the appraisal or professional development review, in which the line manager audits achievements against set standards
Internal audit	Provides independent assurance that an organization's risk management, governance and internal control processes are operating effectively. Auditors report to the Board and Senior Management
External audit	Gives opinion on the credibility and reliability of financial reports to the organization's stakeholders. Additionally, external bodies such as the Care Quality Commission (CQC) will audit to ensure that quality standards are met
Continuous audit	Standards are audited continuously
Random audit	Standards are randomly selected and audited
Focused audit	A specific area for audit is chosen
Retrospective audit	Involves audit of medical records once a patient has been discharged
Non-criterion based audit	A broader audit that goes beyond meeting agreed standards

(Sale 2005)

Activity

* Thinking about when you have been involved in audit, which of the approaches above have been utilized by your organization?

Resources

The Healthcare Quality Improvement Partnership (HQIP) was established in April 2008 to promote quality in healthcare and thereby increase the impact that clinical audit has on healthcare quality in England and Wales. Guidance, training and support for clinical audit can be accessed at http://www.hqip.org.uk/guidance-support

---

Key point summary

Audit is a quality improvement and a change process based on the appraisal of current practice. It identifies both excellent practice as well as the need to improve practice. Audit sits in the fifth and final stage of the evidence cycle and all health and social care professionals have a duty to conform to the audit process. There are a number of off the shelf audit tools, but in many cases teams will design their own. In the case of designing their own tool, Chambers and Wakley's (2005) protocol may be useful and can be used in conjunction with the audit cycle (figure 8.2). Teams will also have to consider the advantages, disadvantages and barriers to implementing an audit.

Implications for practice

* Audit should be embraced and seen as a part of everyday practice.
* It is essential that you choose the right audit tool to evaluate the quality issue.
* An appropriate audit approach must be selected (table 8.9).
* Recognizing that there are advantages and disadvantages to audit.

End-of-chapter questions

1. What approach would you use when there has been an unexpected outcome to treatment given?
2. When might you undertake a retrospective audit?

3. Name three barriers to clinical audit
4. What are the advantages of audit?

See the Appendix on page 194 for suggested answers to these questions.

References

Anderson DG ABC of audit. Cleveland Vocational Training Scheme. http://www.pdp-toolkit.co.uk (accessed 05.11.2013)

Benjamin A (2008) Audit: How to do it in practice. *British Medical Journal*, 336, 1241–1245

Bristol Royal Infirmary Inquiry (2001) *The report of the public inquiry into children's heart surgery at the Bristol Royal Infirmary 1984–1995: Learning from Bristol.* Bristol: Bristol Royal Infirmary inquiry.

Chambers R and Wakley G (2005) *Clinical audit in primary care: Demonstrating quality and outcomes.* Oxford: Radcliffe

Clouston T and Westcott L (2005) *Working in health and social care: An introduction for allied health professionals.* London: Elsevier Churchill Livingstone

Cowan P (2002) Clinical risk management: The role of clinical audit in risk reduction. *British Journal of Clinical Governance*, 7 (3), 220–223

Darzi A (2008) *High quality care for all: NHS next stage review final report.* London: Department of Health

Denscombe M (2010) *The good research guide: For small-scale social research projects.* Maidenhead: McGraw-Hill

Department of Health (1989) *Working for patients.* London: HMSO (Cm 555)

Department of Health (1998) *A first class service: Quality in the new NHS.* London: Department of Health. Available at http://webarchive.nationalarchives.gov.uk/+/www.dh.gov.uk/en/publicationsandstatistics/publications/publicationspolicyand-guidance/dh_4006902 (accessed 28.01.2014)

Department of Health (2006) *Good doctors, safer patients proposals to strengthen the system to assure and improve the performance of doctors and to protect the safety of patients.* London: HMSO

Department of Health (2007) Trust, assurance and safety: The regulation of health professionals. London: HMSO (Cm 7013)

Dilnawaz M, Mazhar H and Shaikh ZI (2012) Clinical audit: A simplified approach. *Journal of Pakistan Association of Dermatologists*, 22 (4), 358–362

Donabedian A (1966) Evaluating the quality of care. *Milleband Memorial Fund Quarterly*, 44, 166–204

Donnellon K, Hurford G and Cox D (2013) It's good to talk: Auditing clinicians' interactions with patients in a primary care setting. *Clinical Governance: An International Journal*, 18 (3), 220–227

Garg D, Singhal A and Neelam K (2010) Clinical audits by trainee doctors: Obstacles and solutions. *Clinical governance: An International Journal*, 17 (1), 45–53

Goldstone LA, Balt JA and Callier M (1983) *Monitor: An index of the quality of nursing care for acute medical and surgical wards.* Newcastle-upon-Tyne: Polytechnic Products

Hicks C (2004) *Research methods for clinical therapists: Applied project design and analysis.* London: Churchill Livingstone

Johnston G, Crombie JK, Davies HTO, Alder EM and Millard A (2000) Reviewing audit: Barriers and facilitating factors for effective clinical audit. *Quality in Healthcare*, 9, 23–36

Lesnik MJ and Anderson BE (1955) *Nursing practice and the law* (2nd ed.). Philadelphia: Lippincott

McSherry R and Pearce P (2011) *Clinical governance: A guide to implementation for healthcare professionals.* London: Blackwell

Morrell C and Harvey G (1999) *The clinical audit handbook: Improving the quality of healthcare.* Oxford: BailliereTindall

NICE (2002) *Principles of best practice in clinical audit.* Oxford: Radcliffe Medical Press

Paskins Z, John H, Hassel A and Rowe I (2010) The perceived advantage and disadvantages of regional audit: A qualitative study. *Clinical Governance: An International Journal*, 15, 200–209

Phaneuf MC (1976) *The nursing audit: Self-regulation in nursing practice.* New York: Appleton-Century-Crofts

Pickering S and Thompson J (2003) *Clinical governance and best value.* London: Churchill Livingstone

Sale D (2005) *Understanding clinical governance and quality assurance: Making it happen.* Basingstoke: Palgrave Macmillan

Swage T (2004) *Clinical governance in healthcare practice.* London: Butterworth Heinemann

Wandelt MA and Ager JW (1974) *Quality patient care scale.* New York: Appleton-Century-Crofts

Wright J and Hill P (2003) *Clinical governance.* London: Churchill Livingstone

Conclusion

We hope that this book has provided you with a greater insight into the importance of clinical governance and how clinical governance should underpin the practice of everyone working in a healthcare setting, regardless of their role. We all, whether we work at a clinical or non-clinical level, have a responsibility to improve practice continuously and implement the clinical governance agenda.

In the UK, quality of healthcare is still very much a current issue despite regular government involvement since the 1990s, the genesis of clinical governance and the requirement to appoint clinical governance leads. This has been evident in the most recent failings at Mid Staffordshire, which were highlighted in the Francis Report (2013).

The inquiries that we have discussed in this book acknowledge that workloads are heavy, resources are limited and staffing levels are not always at optimum levels. However, this should not allow us to settle into complacency. We acknowledge that the creation of clinical governance leads was an important first step in raising awareness of how the clinical governance agenda could improve the quality of healthcare provision. But what was good enough in the early days of clinical governance is no longer good enough now.

We believe that in order for organizations to become learning organizations, the application of two clinical governance strategies must be at the heart of everyone's practice regardless of their role. These strategies are, first, education and training at the individual, team and organizational levels and secondly, Evidence and Values Based Practice (EBP and VBP).

At the most basic level, organizations have a duty to provide education and training so that individuals have an understanding of how to search for and critique literature relevant to their practice. This can be supported further at the team level through journal clubs and critical incident (including complaints) discussions. At the organizational level, healthcare providers have a responsibility to ensure employees have an understanding of the clinical governance agenda and provide relevant CPD opportunities for all staff, regardless of level. All clinical staff have a responsibility for their clinical practice which requires them to ensure that every clinical interaction is evidence and values based. Healthcare is a very fluid environment that continuously changes, and therefore relying on what has been delivered historically will not always result in the provision of best care for the patient and service user. Encouraging all staff to examine the research literature and discuss this with the patient will result in a service that is EBP and VBP.

We furthermore suggest that healthcare professionals are mindful of the work of Bate and Robert (2007), who posit that service users are engaged both at the micro level (co-designing their healthcare) and empowered at the macro level in co-designing the service.

Staff will also be involved with other aspects of clinical governance, such as risk management (e.g. reporting near misses, raising and escalating concerns – including whistle-blowing), complaints management, audit and re-audit. However, these processes are often initiated and managed by more senior staff, for example the clinical governance lead.

To summarize, much has been done to ensure that clinical governance is at the heart of healthcare practice; however, we believe that a further, and deeper, change in organizational culture and thinking is required. Improving the quality of healthcare provision is the responsibility of all members of staff and not just those with a recognized clinical governance remit. A change of thinking is required whereby transparency, openness and candour become the new mantra for healthcare organizations.

Appendix

Suggested answers to questions posed in chapters

Chapter 1

How does an understanding of the definitions of clinical governance help you develop your practice?

The definitions help you to understand that the clinical governance framework impacts on you, your patients and your practice.

The definitions remind us that clinical governance is multifactorial and is everyone's responsibility, not just your manager's.

We therefore need to be engaged in audit, education and training and CQI.

Knowing that clinical governance is everyone's responsibility. How could you become more proactive in implementing your organization's strategy for quality improvement?

You could begin by accessing your organization's strategy and discussing with your line manager in your PDR. You could also discuss in team meetings.

What is the role of the clinical governance lead in your organization?

How do you feed into this role?

Chapter 2

Does your place of work have clear policies pertaining to all of these issues? Do you know where to find them? Are they written in a language that is useful and meaningful to you?

These may be hard copy or available on line, so do ensure you know how to access them.

If you do not find the language accessible, discuss in your team meetings or with your line manager how this could be resolved.

Which aspects of the clinical governance framework could best be applied to assist with a reduction of incidence?

Using Som's definition of clinical governance, think about input, structure, processes and outcomes.

CQI, education and training, risk management, Evidence Based Practice and audit are key aspects of the clinical governance framework.

Chapter 3

How do quality circles differ from focus groups?

Quality circles come together to discuss particular quality issues and begin to consider potential solutions.

Focus groups do not deliver solutions; they are a means of eliciting views on a particular topic.

Quality circles will result in an action plan; focus groups do not.

Which would appear to be your preferred tool?

This could depend on whether you have a preference for a visual representation of an issue rather than a tabular format.

Chapter 4

What are the main barriers to change?

Resistance to change, disempowerment, uncertainty and loss.

Why does change need to be collaborative?

It is no longer appropriate for healthcare providers to adopt a paternalistic approach to care. Patients who are experts by experience need to be involved in the change process in order to become co-designers of their care.

How do developmental, transitional and transformational change differ?

Developmental: to improve current practice.
Transitional: the implementation of something different.
Transformational: emergence of a new state, unknown until it takes shape.

Chapter 5

What are the key differences between Schein's (2010) levels of culture?	The outside layer (artefacts) is visible unlike values, beliefs and underlying assumptions. Decisions to join an organization might be made on a superficial basis (i.e. artefacts). Values, beliefs and underlying assumptions can be understood only once employed in the organization.
Which is the most inclusive of Handy's (1999) four cultural types?	Person culture.
What is the disadvantage of this cultural type?	This may not be the best culture for a health or social care organization, because it lacks structure. The organization is subservient to the individual.

Chapter 6

What is the key difference between quality assurance and CQI?	Quality assurance is a system whereby all procedures that have been designed and planned are followed. The quality assurance function should continually survey the quality philosophy of the organization. The quality assurance team is responsible for auditing all areas to discover and correct errors. CQI is the planning and execution of a flow of improvement to provide quality care that meets or exceeds expectation.
What is the difference between quality assurance and risk management?	Quality assurance is about focusing on the delivery of quality care based on standards and measurable criteria. QA focuses on problem identification, problem assessment, corrective action, follow-up and reporting findings. Risk management is the protection of assets and this is managed by risk identification, risk analysis, risk control or treatment and risk financing.
How does a poor complaints system impact on patients, carers and staff?	Distress may be caused if the complaint is not dealt with swiftly, thoroughly and transparently. Dissatisfaction might occur if patients, carers and staff do not know where to find the complaints policy or if it is not written in plain language. Inadequate responses may cause distress and may exacerbate bereavement (Francis Report 2013).

Chapter 7

Why are EBP and VBP essential to clinical practice?	It is essential that all healthcare professionals understand current evidence in order to (a) challenge current outdated practice and (b) ensure that their practice is up to date. The values of patients/service users and carers must be at the heart of everything we do.
What is the difference between an integrated care pathway and a care bundle?	An integrated pathway identifies the steps of a patient's journey and which professional will carry out the task and provide timeframes. Care bundles are a collection of interventions (usually three to five) that may be applied to the management of a particular condition.
When examining your practice, what is the tool to help you ask an answerable question to ensure your practice is evidence-based?	PICO.
What do the letters stand for?	Depending on usage it could be P: Patient or Population I: Intervention or Indicator C: Comparison or Control O: Outcome. Or P: Patient or Population I: Issue C: Context O: Outcome.

Chapter 8

What approach would you use when there has been an unexpected outcome to treatment given?	A critical incident audit.
When might you undertake a retrospective audit?	Often using patient notes, when looking at what has happened in a particular area, for example the number of patient falls in the past six months.

What are the advantages of audit?	Improve patient care. Improve communication across clinical groups. Increase professional satisfaction. Improved administration.
Name three barriers to clinical audit.	Lack of resources; lack of expertise/ advice in design and analysis; difficulties between groups and group members; lack of an overall plan for audit and organizational hindrance.

Index